Praise for *Life Without Diabetes*

"This fine book contains good science, good writing, and good advice in equal measure. It is both fascinating and useful for readers."

—**Matt Ridley**, author of *The Evolution of Everything*

"Professor Taylor's remarkable tenacity in researching the concept that some people are able to put their type 2 diabetes into remission is changing how we think about and treat this pervasive condition."

—**Dr. Elizabeth Robertson**, Director of Research, Diabetes UK

"Roy Taylor and his team at Newcastle University have not only cracked the mystery of what causes type 2 diabetes, the greatest health problem of our time, but shown the world how to get rid of it. This is a terrific book, which will help a huge number of people."

—**Dr. Michael Mosley**

"Fascinating, informative, and, in today's world, important. For anyone with type 2 diabetes, it's a no-brainer—follow Roy's road map and reverse it. And if you haven't got type 2 diabetes—yet—follow Roy's road map and avoid it."

—**Jimmy Nail**

"This is a truly extraordinary book. When a doctor tells us to do something, we all want to know 'what' and 'how,' but perhaps even more importantly over the long run, 'why.' Professor Taylor does a superb job of explaining all three based on fact rather than fiction. He obviously is a talented teacher as well as a gifted communicator. He presents a clear path to a healthy and enjoyable life crafted with insight and compassion. The information in this book has the potential not only to improve the lives of people with type 2 diabetes, but also to help people who currently do not have diabetes never get it. A remarkable achievement."

—**Robert A. Rizza**, MD, Emeritus
Professor of Medicine, Mayo Clinic

"Professor Taylor is internationally renowned for his clinically relevant research in patients with type 2 diabetes. His work has demonstrated that diet-induced weight loss is a potent therapy that can even induce complete remission of type 2 diabetes in many patients. He translates his years of clinical and research experience into a readable and informative book for patients and their families."

—**Samuel Klein**, MD, and **William H. Danforth**,
Professor of Medicine and Nutritional Science,
Washington University School of Medicine

"This book is a must read for anyone to truly understand how excess food and weight gain lead to type 2 diabetes. Its captivating style will instantly hook you! With a practical approach, it offers a fresh view to live better, enjoy life, and defeat diabetes."

—**Kenneth Cusi**, MD, FACP, FACE,
Professor of Medicine, Division of Endocrinology,
Diabetes, and Metabolism, University of Florida

"Professor Taylor provides the most compelling account I have seen of a bold path to reverse type 2 diabetes. This book offers patients something that no other approach provides: hope through self-reliance."

—**Dr. Domenico Accili**, Professor of Medicine, Columbia
University, and director of the Columbia University
Diabetes and Endocrinology Research Center

Life Without Diabetes

Life Without Diabetes

The Definitive Guide to Understanding and Reversing Type 2 Diabetes

ROY TAYLOR

Professor of Medicine and Metabolism
Newcastle University
and
Honorary Consultant Physician
Newcastle upon Tyne Hospitals NHS
Foundation Trust

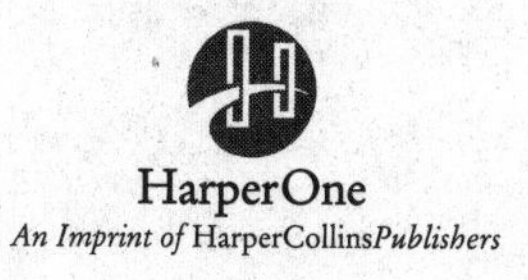

HarperOne
An Imprint of HarperCollins*Publishers*

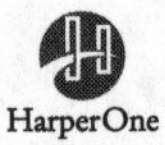

HarperOne

The information contained in this book is provided for general purposes only. It is not intended as and should not be relied upon as medical advice. The publisher and authors are not responsible for any specific health needs that may require medical supervision. If you have underlying health problems or have any questions about the advice contained in this book, you should contact a qualified medical, dietary, or other appropriate professional.

Recipe picture section: photography by Steven Joyce, food styling by Sian Henley, props by Lauren Law.

HarperCollins books may be purchased for educational, business, or sales promotional use. For information, please email the Special Markets Department at SPsales@harpercollins.com.

Originally published as *Life Without Diabetes* in Great Britain in 2019 by Short Books, Unit 316, ScreenWorks, 22 Highbury Grove, London, N5 2ER.

First HarperCollins edition published in 2020.

Library of Congress Cataloging-in-Publication Data has been applied for.

ISBN 978-0-06-293812-1

20 21 22 23 24 LSC 10 9 8 7 6 5 4 3 2 1

This book is dedicated to my patients and research volunteers, who taught me so much

Contents

Foreword by Professor KGMM Alberti

Senior Research Investigator, Imperial College, London UK; previously President, European Association for the Study of Diabetes and International Diabetes Federation

Type 2 diabetes has reached pandemic proportions worldwide. In 1980, we estimated that there were fewer than 100 million people affected—but since then numbers have increased year by year so that we are now heading for 450 million plus, with as many again at high risk. No populations have been spared but figures are particularly high among countries in the Middle East and South Asians.

What is the cause? The big increase has been related to the epidemic of obesity, lack of exercise, and adoption of "modern" nutrition against a genetic susceptibility background. But the precise cause has not previously been identified. Indeed, when WHO reclassified types of diabetes in 1979, type 2 diabetes was diagnosed by exclusion: it was what was left over after type 1 diabetes and other types with known causes were excluded. It was anticipated that the number of people in the type 2 category would fall as specific causes were found. However, in the intervening 40 years one could cynically suggest that not too much has changed. There has been a massive hunt for responsible genes with only limited success. The association with overweight/obesity has certainly been strengthened, although many people with type 2 diabetes are not particularly overweight. Otherwise, it has been a slightly gloomy picture particularly for those who have the disorder. There has also been the view that it is in most people an irreversible disorder.

Professor Taylor in this book shows that the situation is more optimistic. With appropriate food habits and weight loss diabetes *can* be reversed in many people. This is encouraging for the many who have tried but failed due to lack of support and appropriate advice. Even more important, he has identified the key role that fat deposits in the liver and pancreas are fundamental to the development of type 2 diabetes, explaining its hallmarks of diminished insulin secretion and insulin resistance.

The book has something for everyone and is written in an engaging style. There is an excellent exposé of how metabolism works and how glucose is made and used, and how this all goes wrong in type 2 diabetes. He then goes on to show how it can be controlled or indeed reversed by sensible lifestyle and diet choices. It is eminently readable and suitable for anyone with an interest, be they people with diabetes, those with diabetes in the family, anyone curious as to what happens to food in their body, or health care professionals. The book breaks new ground and is a compelling and instructive read.

How to Use This Book

Some books are to be swallowed whole, others to be browsed or enjoyed in part.

For people with type 2 diabetes who wish to escape without delay, Chapter 7 might be where it is opened. For anyone interested in how the body normally copes with food and what goes wrong to cause the metabolic mayhem of type 2 diabetes, Chapters 1 to 6 come first. For people in a hurry, the essence of the book can be picked up in minutes by reading the Quick Read boxes at the end of each chapter, and maybe looking at the pictures.

But if you would like to read a story of scientific adventure, and understand how your body deals with food, then the Lewis Carroll approach is for you: start at the beginning, go on to the end, then stop.

The book provides information but not personal medical advice. If you are already on treatment for diabetes, do discuss with your doctor or diabetes nurse before making changes.

Introduction

Seven days? Just seven days to slay the monster?

For centuries, doctors have regarded type 2 diabetes as a lifelong disease. A disease that can cause great misery—threats to eyesight, to limbs, to the heart—and one that just gets worse and worse, needing more and more tablets and eventually insulin. The moment your doctor says, "You have diabetes," life changes. It is a hammer blow. Your health suddenly appears very fragile. The future is uncertain.

But suddenly, there on the page was a potential breakthrough—the final piece of a jigsaw puzzle that made type 2 diabetes look simple and reversible. It was 2006 and I was sitting just where I am now, at my desk. Reading scientific journals and keeping up with the latest information about diabetes is part of my job, and I had just turned over a page in one of the leading diabetes publications. The graph hit me between the eyes.

It showed what happened to blood sugar in the days immediately after bariatric surgery in people with type 2 diabetes. The graph line plunged from the usual high level on the day before surgery all the way down to absolutely normal by day seven. Normal blood sugar levels? In seven days? That had never been seen before. No other treatment could achieve this dramatic normalization. All the research of the previous few decades seemed to come together in a flash. But could it be true?

But this story really starts in 1970, when as a student at Edinburgh Medical School I attended a series of lectures by Professor Reginald Passmore, in which he explained physiology as a sequence of logical thoughts. Physiology is the science of how the body works. I can still see his tall, lean frame topped with gray hair as he laid out clear lines of reasoning—always with a dry sense of humor. I was riveted as he demonstrated that commonly accepted "knowledge" could be reassessed by clear thinking and using solid information about how things work. How certain or uncertain could we be about common beliefs? This was exciting. Suddenly, "facts" could be seen to be merely links of varying reliability. Anything could and should be reexamined in the light of new information. After all, Newton seemed to be conclusively correct about his laws of motion and gravity from the 17th century onwards, but Einstein showed that they were not exactly correct. In turn, current knowledge shows that Einstein was not entirely correct either—subatomic particles do not obey the theory of relativity.

But Passmore will be forever correct in having taught that knowledge should be continually reassessed, especially in supporting medical decisions, where any part of the accepted framework of facts must remain open to repeated scrutiny as new concepts emerge.

Skip on a few years and, as a newly qualified doctor, I became fascinated by the way in which all the hormones in our bodies work together to help control our health, and in particular by the fact that the hormone insulin doesn't function properly in people with type 2 diabetes. I spent a number of years trying to understand the link between insulin and diabetes. During this time I continued to work as a doctor, mainly dealing with medical emergencies as they came into the hospital, but gradually specializing more and more in diabetes.

In 2006, I had just brought together, as part of a multi-million-pound research project at Newcastle University, brilliant physicists with state-of-the-art scanners to create the Newcastle Magnetic Resonance Centre. The idea was to develop new techniques to look at any organ in the body, but of course my interest was to investigate the main organs involved with diabetes. And it was not long after we had established the center that I experienced the eureka moment—that graph with its new concept that high blood sugar levels in type 2 diabetes could be normalized in seven days. By coincidence, we were in a perfect position to carry out the breakthrough studies described in this book.

By 2011, we were able to publish the scientific proof that type 2 diabetes was reversible, and within five years to confirm the "how" and the "why" of this apparent impossibility. Both the initial proof and the follow-up studies were based on the amazing story of how the body manages energy from food.

You will remember snippets from your school biology lessons. The heart pumps blood around the body, the lungs enable us to take in oxygen and get rid of carbon dioxide. But there is one dynamic function, absolutely key to the maintenance of a healthy body, of which most people are totally unaware: what happens to food after it leaves the gut. How is the energy supply managed? All will be explained.

Ask someone what type 2 diabetes is and they are likely to tell you that the disease is something to do with too much sugar. It is true that diabetes occurs when there is excess glucose in the bloodstream—with devastating effects on the eyes, feet, heart and brain. However, my research has shown that type 2 diabetes is caused by just one factor: too much fat in the liver and pancreas. In the normal functioning of the body, the pancreas produces insulin to help the liver control the supply of glucose to the rest of the body. When there is excess fat in the liver, however, it responds poorly to insulin, produces too much glucose, and passes on excess fat to the pancreas. As a result of that, the insulin-producing cells of the pancreas cease to function properly.

It is important to say that you don't have to be obese, or even look overweight, to have type 2 diabetes. Every individual has their "personal fat threshold"—the point at which no more can be taken into their regular fat cells (in the fatty layer under the skin, especially around the thighs and trunk). The fat has to go somewhere, and it ends up not only inside the tummy cavity but also inside the main organs of the body. If the insulin-secreting cells in the pancreas are susceptible to fat-induced problems, this is the tipping point for diabetes. This susceptibility is just the luck of the draw, depending on your genes.

My goal in this book is to make the new understanding

of type 2 diabetes accessible to all. And by doing so, to help people with this devastating condition, and their families, to deal with it as effectively as possible. Drawing on the latest experimental insights, I will offer a definitive account of how type 2 diabetes develops. Along the way, I will explain the workings of your body and show how our modern lifestyle has interfered with the beautifully balanced processes evolved over millennia.

There is a surprisingly simple solution. One that most definitely involves weight loss, but which is not really about a diet. The word "diet" is enough to put anyone off. It tends to be associated with an unpalatable change to eating and (usually) a failure to bring about desired weight change. Our original approach to these problems in Newcastle recognized that two very different phases were required: first, a step change in weight and then, a long-term way of living. In our very first study we also learned that an additional phase, a gradual, managed transition between these two phases, was helpful.

I initially came up with the weight loss method simply as a research tool to allow us to study the changes that occurred when people with diabetes potentially became normal again. It was a means of understanding the cause of type 2 diabetes. This pragmatic way of losing weight, based mainly on complete nutrition drinks, proved highly effective. And surprisingly, our volunteers actually found the approach acceptable and nowhere near as difficult as they had thought. Most of them lost 15kg (about 33 lbs) in eight weeks and felt really well. Before we knew it, the "Newcastle Diet," as people spontaneously started calling it, took on a life of its own. It is a basic recipe for success—for anyone who really wants be rid of type 2 diabetes.

I hope this book will explain to anyone with type 2 diabetes how it may be possible to return to full health. I will also offer practical and validated advice on how to enjoy life while remaining free of the disease. I want every reader to come away with an understanding of how the body handles food, what goes wrong in the case of what we now know to be a relatively simple disease, and what must be done in order to escape from its clutches.

1

What Is Type 2 Diabetes?

A Snake in the Grass

Diabetes is a condition that slowly attacks important parts of the body—without warning.

The process happens over many years and during this time people may feel perfectly well. However, silently, stealthily, high glucose levels are stacking up problems, and serious consequences then often appear suddenly, at which point it can be difficult to return to full health. Doctors refer to these as "complications" of diabetes, a polite term that underplays the awfulness for the person concerned. However, once you know that there is a snake hidden in the grass, and that it is very venomous, you can minimize the chance of being bitten.

The good news is that the risk of developing these long-term problems can be decreased by controlling the level of blood glucose as well as possible. The better news is that if blood glucose is returned to normal, then the risk of damage to eyes, nerves, feet, kidneys, heart, and brain returns to the same level as for people of similar age and weight without diabetes. From the point of view of the person staring down the barrel of a gun, that is a miracle. Explaining this miracle is the main purpose of this book.

Sugar and Diabetes

Diabetes just means the level of sugar in the blood is too high.

What exactly is sugar? The word covers any sweet, simple form of carbohydrate. The sugar in your blood is a particular kind called glucose. Ordinary table sugar is made up of two kinds of sugar bound together. Half is glucose and the other half is fructose (which is a very similar sugar commonly found in fruit). But the kind of sugar does not matter, as your body will convert the fructose to glucose as needed. Glucose is the basic form of sugar that your body uses for energy.

In healthy people, blood glucose levels are very tightly controlled. Overnight, this control happens minute by minute to keep levels constant. Even after a birthday banquet, the increase in blood glucose is quite small. This is achieved by a huge and rapid increase in the blood level of insulin, the main hormone that controls blood glucose. If this mechanism breaks down, blood glucose rises too much after eating.

Does this matter? Sugar looks so innocent, sitting there in the sugar bowl, so ubiquitous in our lives today that it may be difficult to imagine that it was once a luxury item, with the supply of honey from monasteries being the only source of added sweetness to food. We have become accustomed to it being added to almost everything. But, yes, it does matter, because if the glucose levels in blood become too high, problems will occur throughout the body.

This book is all about type 2 diabetes, which is by far the commonest form of the disease. The other types each have a very different cause (take a look at the Appendix for details). But all forms result in high blood glucose levels and can cause similar long-term complications. Being sure that a person has one type of diabetes rather than another is not easy. Around 90% of people found to have high blood glucose have type 2. And if you have put on weight in adult life, are over 30 years old, and have high blood sugars, it is highly likely that you have type 2 rather than one of the other forms.

But there is no test that can definitively confirm this diagnosis and the other types of diabetes can sometimes be mistaken for type 2. It is up to the doctor to consider whether one of the other types could be the correct diagnosis.

If you or someone close to you has type 2 diabetes, you will probably have a lot of questions. What will it do to me? Is it the serious kind? How can I control my blood sugar levels? Let's look at these and some other key concerns surrounding the disease.

Why Do Glucose Levels Shoot Up After Meals?

As soon as the first mouthful of a meal is swallowed, it is broken down in the stomach and glucose is rapidly released from it into the blood. For instance, from an average helping of pasta with vegetables, digestion releases about 30 teaspoonfuls of sugar. To deal with this sudden unleashing of glucose, the body normally responds by rapidly increasing insulin levels. And, if the right amount of insulin is made, blood glucose levels are quickly brought under control. However, if this does not happen, they rise rapidly.

The pancreas—specifically, the beta cells in the pancreas—should provide this insulin, but if they are not working properly or are compromised in some way, they fail to make enough at the right time and diabetes develops. To make matters worse in type 2 diabetes, the body does not respond well to whatever insulin is on offer. The levels of insulin in the blood may slowly creep up, but even at very high levels the job still can't be done. And so blood glucose levels rise and rise after meals—and then take hours to decrease.

Why Is My Glucose Level High Before Breakfast?

If you have diabetes, you may be puzzled that your blood glucose is high first thing in the morning—after the overnight fast. Why is it high even though no food has been eaten for 12 hours or more? Sometimes this "fasting" glucose level is even higher than it was at bedtime. What is going on? Surely you didn't go sleepwalking to the fridge?

To answer this question, we first need to understand the neat way that fasting blood glucose is normally controlled. First thing in the morning, none of the glucose molecules in your blood have come directly from food. The last meal is a distant metabolic memory. In fact, virtually all your blood glucose has been made by your own body; by your liver. Why does your body make this toxic stuff? Well, because a constant level of glucose is necessary for life (we will go into this further in Chapters 3 and 4). We need it to fuel the brain and as a potential instant source of energy for muscles—so that we are braced for action at all times, even when we are woken up suddenly and have to run away from danger. The key word is "constant": glucose easily passes from the bloodstream into the tissues of the body, and because it can be toxic, its production is normally tightly regulated. In type 2 diabetes this regulation is lost, and your liver makes glucose too enthusiastically.

What Is the Usual Treatment for Type 2 Diabetes?

Official guidelines for the treatment of type 2 diabetes lay out a depressing prospect of steadily increasing numbers of tablets, then injections, then insulin treatment. A person newly diagnosed with type 2 diabetes has a 50:50 chance of being on insulin injections within 10 years.

The first thing a person with diabetes is told is that they should lose weight and take more exercise. All too often, this message is recited without any conviction that it will be effective or any information on how it can be achieved. You may be given a "diet sheet," even though it is known that this is ineffective by itself. But often, the immediate next step is to be prescribed a tablet—to help keep your blood glucose down. This will usually be metformin. Metformin is cheap, comes in the size of a horse pill, and has "side effects."

The term "side effects" is a marvelous medical euphemism for things that trouble the patient but not the doctor. The important thing, as far as a doctor or nurse is concerned, is that the prescribed tablet has the desired effect—i.e., to control your blood glucose. Side effects are simply to be tolerated. "But Doctor, I can't go out for fear of needing the bathroom quickly." Perhaps we should revise the words and talk about the *total effects* of a drug—after all, you are the expert on what is happening to your body.

One good thing about metformin is that it does not cause further weight gain. Another good thing is that it only pushes blood glucose down if the level is high, and it does not cause troublesome episodes of low blood glucose known as hypos. From the medical point of view, it is a relatively safe drug in most people.

But metformin has only a modest effect on blood glucose control and after a while additional medication will be required. The cheaper options, such as gliclazide, glibenclamide, and gliquidone, all cause weight gain, as well as sudden dizziness if your glucose levels get too low (i.e., a hypo). More expensive options (e.g., pioglitazone) do not cause hypos, but pile on the weight and they may make your ankles swell. The most expensive newer options (gliptins or gliflozins) do neither of these things but have other side effects. For a proportion of people, having to take tablets is undesirable for very good reasons.

Once you are taking two or three different tablets and your glucose levels are still uncontrolled, an injection may be recommended. Liraglutide and drugs like it are very different from insulin. Basically, what these drugs do is dramatically slow down the rate at which the stomach empties after a meal, thus preventing food, and particularly glucose, from getting into the body too fast. They also have the really useful effect of limiting the amount of food you eat, as your stomach feels full sooner. Some people vomit or feel nauseous when they start this treatment—but don't worry, it is only a side effect!

And then there is insulin. In many people, insulin can improve the control of blood glucose modestly, but the devil is in the detail of a particular side effect—the hypos. You may find your blood glucose is pushed too low in an entirely unpredictable manner. This can cause all kinds of problems in day-to-day life—for instance when driving, climbing up ladders, or just pottering around the kitchen. The driving implications are serious, and when you first go on insulin your driving license has to be changed to one that has to be renewed every three years. As if this was not bad enough, most people put on more weight after being started on insulin.

"Treatment" is another word that is open to interpretation. When a patient asks, "Can my diabetes be treated, Doctor?" they want to know whether treatment can restore normality, as with antibiotics for an infection, or a plaster cast for a broken bone. But what the doctor tends to hear is "Are there guidelines on treatment with drugs for this condition?" and so answers "Yes." There are plenty of official guidelines. But neither the small effect of these in making things better, nor the likely litany of future health problems gets much of a mention.

The good news that type 2 diabetes can be "treated" conveys the wrong message to many people and creates a false sense of security. This is exacerbated by the tendency of well-meaning official information sites to make light of the reality of the condition, emphasizing that life can continue pretty much as normal with it. The uncomfortable truth is not stated—that the main complications are only somewhat mitigated and that even the best conventional treatments do not eliminate the considerable risk of future health problems.

I Am Not Obese So Why Do I Have Type 2 Diabetes?

Contrary to popular opinion, type 2 diabetes actually has very little to do with obesity—although it does concern weight, and more specifically whether you are overweight *for you*.

Today, the steadily increasing average weight means

that there are of course more people who are very heavy or "morbidly obese." With media attention focusing upon this very serious condition in any discussion of weight, you'd be forgiven for thinking it was the main problem. But in fact, the elephant in the room is not the number of very heavy people. It is the vast majority who are just heavier than would be ideal.

The trouble is that many people regard themselves as being of normal weight because they are similar to the majority of other people of the same age. But the word "normal" has a double meaning here. If a person is within the range typical of the population, they can be said to be normal. But that is not necessarily healthy or ideal.

Are you the same weight as you were when you were 25 years old? Just look at folk on the main street. People aged around 20 years tend to be slimmer than those aged around 60 years. In Western society we gain around half a kilogram a year through most of our adult life. This is not to do with aging or with hormones—it simply reflects the environment we live in. And that environment is setting up a time bomb. In the UK, even though people aged 20 tend to be slimmer than those aged 60, young people too are heavier than ever before, and over one third start adult life far too heavy. As a group, it is certain that they will get type 2 diabetes at a younger age than their parents. This time bomb deserves a book to itself.

There is no biological reason why people need to put on weight during adult life. In societies where food is not a heavily promoted pastime, and it is necessary to walk or cycle for everyday business, body weight tends to remain much more stable as people age. But obviously, in the consumerist environment we inhabit in the developed world, where enticing, quick-fix, calorie-dense food is everywhere and heavily marketed, you actually have to be unusually disciplined (or just not that bothered by food) to avoid putting on weight.

Societal perceptions are important in all this. And for much of my career as a doctor and academic I have been pondering these and how we might agree to change them. Perhaps TV and film producers could move toward avoiding the usual stereotypes? Certainly, this issue deserves wide discussion.

Food for Diabetes or Diabetic Food?

Part of the treatment for type 2 involves adjusting the kinds of foods eaten. In chemists and in supermarkets, you may see on the shelves "diabetic foods." Typically, these products are made with sugars that are more slowly and incompletely absorbed, such as sorbitol. However, such foods contain at least as many calories as their less expensive, ordinary equivalents. They do not make a worthwhile difference to blood glucose control and certainly do not help with weight loss. All doctors and health professionals now discourage the use of diabetic foods, because they do not help. People with diabetes need just the same fuels for everyday life as the rest of the population, and far more effective than eating special foods is simply cutting back on both sugar and calorie consumption.

It is certainly true that what and how much you eat can modify how well you control your blood glucose. Guidelines are steadily changing toward the rational approach of avoiding high-sugar foods and too much carbohydrates, but information sources offer varying advice and few emphasize the central importance of limiting the total *quantity* of food. Magazines and newspapers frequently carry advice that is misleading.

What do you eat? In everyday life, most people eat what their family or friends eat. It can be a challenge to change family habits but small adjustments can make a big difference. For instance, halving your portion of potato/pasta/rice and doubling your serving of vegetables would be good. There are plenty more ideas later in the book about how to set in place better eating habits.

Living with the Immediate Problems of Type 2 Diabetes

If you found out about your diabetes after a visit to the doctor prompted by troublesome symptoms, then you will already know about some of the problems the condition causes.

When blood glucose levels go too high, glucose starts spilling into the urine. And, because glucose draws water along with it, this causes the kidneys to make more urine than usual. In people without diabetes, the kidneys keep all the glucose in the blood, and do not waste any of it in urine. As the descendants of people who survived famine after famine over millennia, we have evolved to be energy-efficient. Losing energy obtained from food would be a problem. But when presented with an overwhelming amount of glucose, the poor old kidneys cannot cope. They have not evolved to deal with that.

If you have diabetes, passing large volumes of urine will be all too familiar. If your diabetes is out of control—perhaps if you've eaten too much or forgotten your tablets or injections—passing too much urine is a sure sign that blood glucose has become too high. It's likely that you will have to get up in the night to go to the toilet more often. Also, because water is being lost from the body, you will feel thirsty and so find yourself wanting to drink a lot of fluids. This might have been one of the warning symptoms announcing the presence of your diabetes; however, because the threshold for spilling glucose into the urine varies so much between individuals, other problems may have occurred first.

For instance, you may have been generally out of sorts or tired. Of course, fatigue can be caused by many things, so if other symptoms have not occurred, a link with diabetes may not have immediately been made. But it is often the start of a catalogue of problems. Among the commonest problems leading to a diagnosis of diabetes are infections of the skin. Other life forms like to feed on glucose, and they set up house wherever easy pickings are to be had. Itchiness and inflammation of the penis or vulva can result from candida infections. But any sort of bacterial infection is more likely when blood glucose levels are raised. Breaks in the skin—small cuts or other trivial injuries—are prone to get infected, and urine infections are very common. This may sound like a depressing list—but that is not the worst of it.

This section has described only the immediate consequences. If blood glucose levels are raised for years, then more serious longer-term problems may start stacking up.

The Longer-Term Problems of Type 2 Diabetes

All your organs depend upon food and oxygen delivered by the blood, and, as these have to reach every cell of the body, you have a fine network of capillaries throughout every organ. These delicate blood vessels are very good at delivering the goods right to where they are needed. We all depend upon them absolutely. But they are highly sensitive to raised blood glucose levels. Over a long time, high levels of glucose can cause capillaries to become inefficient, leaky, or simply blocked. And, when cells don't get their regular grocery order, trouble occurs throughout the body.

The eye is particularly sensitive. The back of the eye, the retina, depends upon a very efficient network of capillaries supplying the light-sensitive nerve endings. If these capillaries start leaking, fluid collects in the retina and can threaten eyesight. If capillaries within the retina become blocked, the light-sensitive nerves cannot work properly. Diabetes is a major cause of sight loss. In fact, before effective eye screening, it was the commonest preventable cause of blindness in the UK.

Nerves elsewhere in the body are affected too, as they need food and oxygen to conduct messages. Have you ever experienced a "dead-leg"? By sitting awkwardly and squeezing a nerve for too long you will have blocked the capillary flow of blood to the nerve and caused it to stop working. You will have felt numbness and tingling and been unable to make your muscles do what you want them to. Fortunately, this is rectified within a few minutes of relieving the pressure. But nerve problems in diabetes are not so easily reversed, following as they do from years of capillary damage. Numbness, tingling, and even pain can last for months and may become permanent. As the nerves to the feet are the longest in the body, numbness is commonest there. And this numbness is a big problem in itself, because it prevents the body's normal means of alerting us to trouble—i.e., feeling pain. If your new shoes are rubbing, you will stop walking or change shoes. But if you cannot feel the pain, you will carry on walking while the damage continues silently. This can lead to skin breaking down and open the door to infections, the poor blood supply caused by damaged capillaries allowing bacteria to spread unchecked with potentially devastating consequences. The motto for feet in diabetes is "check 'em or lose 'em." That may sound brutal, but there is no point in my putting a gloss on things here: providing clear information about the very real risks is essential. You do not want a doctor who will cover up the actuality. In the UK today, about 170 amputations are performed every week because of diabetes. Yes, *every week*.

Larger blood vessels can be affected, as well as the

capillaries. They become more easily blocked by fatty changes in the vessel wall and, as you may know, blockages in the blood vessels supplying the heart cause heart attacks, while blockages in those supplying the brain cause strokes. This is why heart attacks and strokes are more common in people with diabetes. Meanwhile, blockages in the main blood vessels in the legs cause poor circulation to the feet, making other problems worse, and amputation more likely.

High glucose levels can also cause the kidneys not just to struggle but to lose function altogether. Once beyond the earliest stages, this loss of function is genuinely irreversible and seriously impairs health. Diabetes accounts for around half of those needing kidney dialysis treatment three times every week. That does not lead to a great quality of life.

The likelihood of serious complications as a result of type 2 diabetes depends quite a lot on your age. Perhaps counterintuitively, the younger you are at the time of diagnosis, the greater the risk of serious trouble. A young person getting type 2 diabetes faces much higher risks of serious illness than does a person of the same age getting type 1 diabetes and needing insulin injections. A 45-year-old man newly diagnosed with diabetes has a more than 50% chance of not being able to work until the age of 65 because of heart attacks, stroke, or serious foot problems. And that 45-year-old man will lose an average of six years of life. Whereas, for anyone who is diagnosed over the age of 70 years, the chance of major health problems remains similar to people of the same age without diabetes.

Annual Checks

One of the triumphs of modern diabetes management in the UK (and some other countries) is that the main curse of the disease—loss of eyesight—has been lifted. When I was appointed as consultant in 1985, there were six people under the age of 25 years in my clinic who were registered as blind due to diabetes. Today there are none, largely because annual checks using a simple, effective test have become part of routine health care in the UK since the 1980s. If picked up early enough, deterioration can be prevented by specialist eye treatment for most people.

Also, present-day knowledge about blood pressure in diabetes has led to early treatment being widely advised. It is now relatively simple to reduce blood pressure to acceptable levels—unlike blood glucose. And active treatment of blood pressure has had a big effect, in particular, on decreasing the chance of glucose-induced kidney failure. A simple annual urine test gives a good early warning of any trouble.

Another important element of treatment these days is the advice to take off your shoes, at least once a year! Your doctor or nurse (or podiatrist if available) needs to check that your nerves are working well enough for you to feel possible danger. Similarly, the circulation of blood to your feet needs to be checked. Simple and effective action can be taken if problems are detected. Feet tend to be the most neglected part of the body and are the butt of comedians' jokes. But these remarkable organs should be appreciated. Have a look at yours. What amazing works of engineering! As you step forward, your forefoot, without any complaint, bears about one and a half times your body weight. Well worth checking. Well worth looking after.

Nevertheless, while the introduction of the annual review visit has been successful in decreasing serious problems for people with diabetes, how much better it would be to prevent any problems occurring at all—by reversing your diabetes altogether!

I hope this chapter has clarified a few of the myths and misunderstandings that tend to flourish around type 2 diabetes and its treatment. I'm going to go on to explain why you get the condition and what you can do about it. But in order to do that effectively we first need to consider how the body works and how it converts food into fuel…

Quick Read

- Diabetes means that blood glucose is higher than normal
- Type 2 diabetes is caused by the insulin-producing cells of the pancreas not working normally
- It is made worse by the body not responding normally to insulin
- The immediate problems associated with the condition tend to be thirst, passing

too much urine, and tiredness; but the long-term complications can be extremely serious

- Conventional treatment of diabetes, including an annual review, does decrease the risk of complications, but only moderately

2

Energy for Life: The Dual Fuel

Greetings, carbon-based biped!

These words by Arthur C. Clarke hit the nail on the head: beings from outer space would probably be amused by the idea of bodies moving around on two legs, and fascinated to discover that we get our energy from the element carbon. On earth, all known life forms are based on carbon. All our food energy comes from carbon. Each unit of glucose is a string of six carbon atoms; each unit of fat is made up of strings of 40–60 linked carbon atoms. Such is the beautiful simplicity of the basics of life. That is what this chapter is all about.

To be more precise, the energy that we rely on is actually stored in the links *between* carbon atoms. Just as a fire releases energy as heat from the carbon in wood, our bodies obtain the energy from the carbon links in foods. A fire needs oxygen to carry away waste carbon in smoke as the gas carbon dioxide. In just the same way, your body needs oxygen to carry away waste carbon—also in the form of carbon dioxide. You simply breathe it out via your lungs, not noticing that these carbon atoms entered your body as a potato. Or a lentil. Or an olive. You no longer need the carbon, because your body has cleverly extracted the energy that was tied up in those chemical links between the carbon atoms in foods. And because that chemical energy is released partly as heat, your body is warm to the touch.

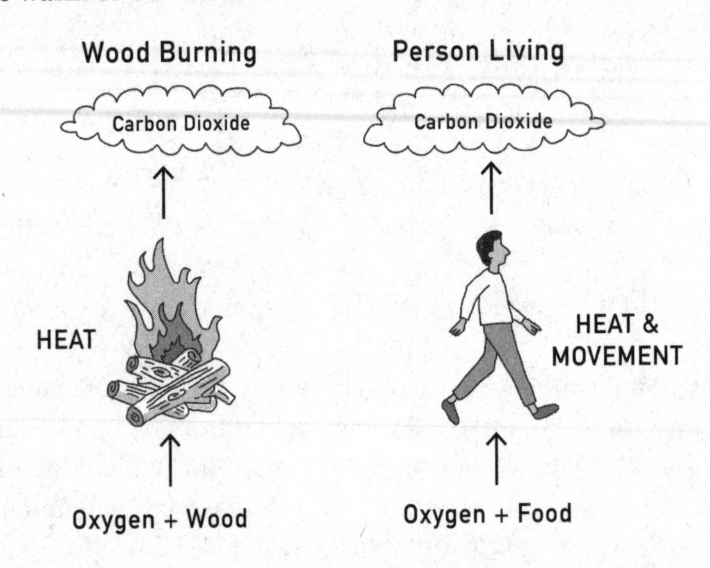

2.1 A fire releases energy as heat from the links between carbon atoms in wood. The waste carbon is carried away in smoke. The human body releases energy to use for both heat and movement from the links between carbons in food. The waste carbon is breathed out as carbon dioxide.

Like animals, plants need to generate and store energy. This happens at a basic level as plants forge chemical links by building up carbon chains using sunlight energy. To do this, they take up carbon dioxide from the air and link the carbons to create high-energy sugars or fats.

Plants conveniently store these, and in turn we might eat them—perhaps as potatoes, rice, or cassava—or, equally, a farmer might feed them to other animals, to promote a concentration of energy in milk or meat.

The bottom line is that, whether we are eating animals or vegetables, food provides us with carbon-based energy that allows us to live and work and play. Our bodies merely need to direct the right amounts of food energy to storage and the right amount to releasing the essential energy, second by second and minute by minute.

Just Ticking Over

We don't expect machines to run without fuel. You would not get far in your car without it. The human body is no different, and an average person may use around 2,400 calories of energy per day. Even if you are reading this lying in bed completely relaxed, your body is using energy just to stay alive. Your heart works constantly, pumping blood around the body. Every cell in your body is continuously busy, pumping out substances it doesn't need and pumping in others. The liver in particular is busy—manufacturing whatever sort of fuel the body requires at this moment in time. It can make glucose from substances released from elsewhere in the body—for instance, from lactic acid (a string of three carbons) or the components of any protein surplus to requirements. If there is too much glucose around, the liver can turn it into fat. The liver never rests.

Staying alive demands a lot of energy and we have evolved ways of building up reserves whenever possible. What if you were snowed in and your cupboards were bare? Or shipwrecked on a desert island? This would not cause a problem for your clever body, or at least not for several weeks. The only daily essential is water.

That said, big creatures require more energy than small creatures to stay alive. How much energy you need when lying down depends upon your size. If two dogs are snoozing peacefully in front of the fire, the St. Bernard is burning much more energy than the Chihuahua. The person paying for the dog food may well have guessed this.

For humans, the amount of energy the resting body needs every minute can be measured directly. The graph below shows results from a large number of people and demonstrates how the need for energy increases steadily as weight increases. It also shows how the need for energy decreases if weight decreases.

Imagine a person weighing 154 pounds lying perfectly still. On average, for each kilogram of body weight in a woman, just under one calorie is needed every minute. For the whole 154 pounds body, 60 calories are used every hour to power the vital processes of life. Over a 24-hour period of lying completely still, that amounts to 1,450 calories being required. Whereas for a woman weighing 220 pounds, 1.2 calories are required every minute, or about 1,770 calories in the 24-hour period.

The average man requires slightly more energy due to

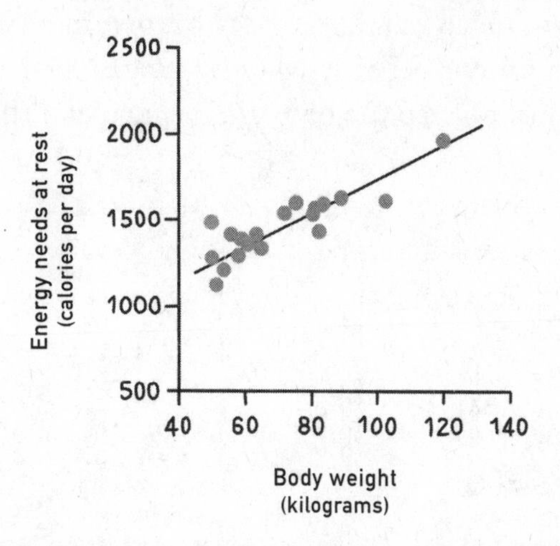

2.2 Energy needs—bigger people need more to keep weight steady.

his typically different body composition, but the effect of body size is just the same. A 154-pound man will burn around 1,500 calories at rest in 24 hours, while a 220-pound man will require almost 25% more (around 1,900 calories). Of course, these are average numbers and individuals may need more or less.

Exercise Versus Activity

Everyone expects that the body will need more energy if it is moving around. And to some extent, this is true. But the actual amount of energy spent during exercise is much smaller than most people imagine. The diagram below shows how much extra energy is burned in a half-hour period of various activities. For comparison, the energy required just to keep the body ticking over is also shown.

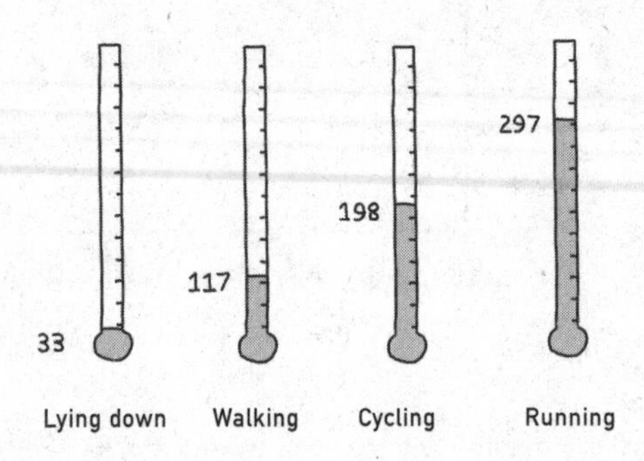

2.3 How many calories are burned in half an hour? The numbers shown are for a woman weighing 176 pounds, during moderately brisk walking, cycling, and running.

Fred and Bill are neighbors and both weigh 220 pounds. Fred wants to lose a few pounds, so he dusts off his squash racquet and after a slow start settles into playing for half an hour on Saturday mornings. Bill enjoys puttering around his garden. He steadily trims, weeds, and sorts, never out of breath. One Saturday morning, rather red in the face, Fred leans over the fence and tells Bill that he ought to take some exercise. But then Fred finds that his own weight does not decrease, so he builds up even more of a sweat during his half-hour on the squash court. Who burns more energy each Saturday morning?

The answer lies in the *time* that the body is burning

more than the resting level. For the half-hour on the court, Fred increases his energy usage from 1.3 calories each minute to an average of eight calories each minute. In half an hour he burns 240 calories. But then he sits down to recover and reads the paper for the rest of the morning, feeling good. In the next three and a half hours, staying seated, he burns 315 calories. Each Saturday morning a total of 555 calories are burned.

Bill meanwhile walks around his garden, moving this and that and trimming here and there. He is active for four hours—three and a half hours longer than Fred—and expends more energy without breaking a sweat. Staying on his feet, carrying his 220 pounds around, he uses an average of 2.5 calories per minute—600 calories in all, which is 45 more than Fred. And, for Fred, there is a further snag. On leaving his squash club, he has to walk past the vending machines, and with the glow of righteous exercise, he often treats himself to a little chocolate bar (only 100g), in two minutes flat acquiring another 400 calories.

So it is the *duration* of physical activity rather than the intensity that has more effect in determining how much energy is used. As an extreme example, when Ranulph Fiennes and Mike Stroud walked across Antarctica pulling heavy sledges over mountains and crevasses for up to 14 hours per day, it was estimated that they burned 11,500 calories every day! Gluttons for punishment as they are, even Fiennes and Stroud would not have been able to burn anything like that in shorter bursts of more intense exercise.

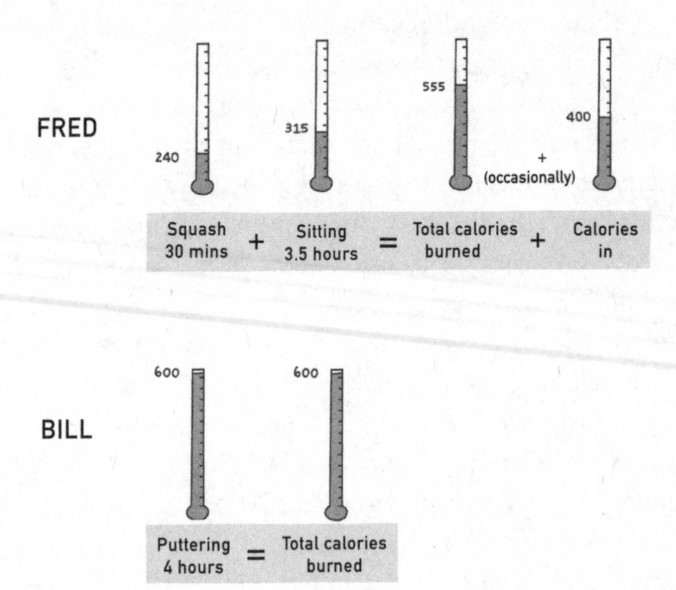

2.4 Number of calories burned on a Saturday morning and why Fred did not lose weight.

If your aim is to prevent weight gain, being moderately active for hours is more effective than a quick burst in the gym. You don't have to take sweaty exercise—although, if your aim is to maximize heart function and fitness, then bursts of additional brisk exercise are important. Advice handed out by exercise experts or public-health doctors tends not to point out the important difference between the very separate aims of cardiovascular fitness and weight control. With his bouts of squash, Fred's heart is likely in better shape than Bill's—but that was not his goal. He started playing again because he wanted to lose a few pounds.

Preventing weight gain is arguably one of the most important issues facing our society today, and one that could certainly be helped by, for example, changing transportation policy to encourage people to be more active and walk or cycle more, along with legislation on food policy. But preventing weight gain is not the same thing as losing weight; getting rid of excess fat that has accumulated over a long period of time requires a different approach, as we shall see.

Suffice to say that the balance between energy burned during exercise—whatever form of activity you engage in—and energy pouring in from food is very unequal. And for people who want to lose weight, the overwhelming priority must be to cut down on the consumption of food and calorie-containing drinks.

Saving Energy for a Rainy Day

Over the long period of our evolution, human beings have had to cope with frequent periods of food shortage. We have had to survive periods of crop failure or runs of bad luck on the hunting front. As a result, we have developed very clever mechanisms for storing food energy.

All our energy comes from food or drink. Although that is a statement of the obvious, it is a good place to start considering energy for life. After food is eaten, it is broken down by digestion to simpler substances. The liver is a factory that turns substances into useful forms. There are only a few sources of food calories: carbohydrates, fat, protein, and alcohol. From your plate to your body, it goes like this:

Carbohydrates—potatoes, pasta, rice, bread, and all sugars: all broken down to **glucose**.
Fat—butter, oils, dairy produce, fat in meat: all broken down to simpler **fats**.
Protein—meat, lentils, nuts, dairy produce: all broken down to the basic building blocks (called amino acids) used for muscle and other tissues. But any surplus is turned into **glucose**.
Alcohol—broken down and stored as **fat**.

If you glance down the list again, you can see that all your food is turned into either glucose or fat. And those fuels are the source of all energy for your body.

So you can now look at your plate in a new light. Carbohydrates are effectively sugar, and fat is fat. Glucose can be stored as glycogen in the liver and muscles, and fat can be stored under the skin. Any excess protein ends up as glucose. Contrary to popular belief, encouraged by advertisements for protein supplements, excess intake of protein does not build huge muscles. Products with exotic-sounding names such as branch chain amino acids and ox protein boost nothing more than wishful thinking. Amino acids are merely the basic building blocks for proteins. In excess, these building blocks are dealt with summarily by the body—the atoms that make them different are lopped off and their carbon skeletons are thrown into the pool to turn into glucose.

What about alcohol? Surely that is a special fuel? Not at all. Alcohol is essentially liquid fat. It contains almost as much energy as fat—seven calories in every gram, compared with nine in each gram of fat. The liver removes the particular atoms that make alcohol different. Alcohol is simply burned—or stored—as fat.

So in terms of both energy storage in the body and energy usage, we can talk about just glucose and fat. That is the beautiful economy of nature.

Energy Metabolism Is Simple

- Only two fuels are burned for energy by your body—glucose and fat. Both can be stored and used when required.
- Protein is broken down into the building blocks our body needs for growth and maintenance. However, in the Western world, we tend to eat more protein than we need and any excess is converted by the body into glucose.
- Alcohol? Ever efficient, the body merely breaks down alcohol then burns it just as though it had been fat.
- Metabolism is simply the coordinated handling of glucose and fat.

Storing Energy as Glucose

Glucose is tricky to store. It attracts water, and therefore tissues storing glucose would quickly become engorged and damaged. So the body has developed an amazing work-around. By linking together glucose molecules in a chain, or polymer (rather like a string of beads), it effectively immobilizes them, holding them ready for use without causing local problems. The glucose is no longer able to attract water and is safe to store inside muscle or liver cells. This concentrated form of glucose is known as glycogen.

Glycogen comes to popular attention most often in relation to long-distance running. Glycogen-loading is what pasta parties before marathons are all about. Take in lots of carbohydrates and fill the tank to maximum. However, in everyday life, the role of glycogen stores is to help the body control blood glucose after meals. Here's how: after eating a meal, blood glucose levels rise, and the body goes to work removing absorbed glucose from the blood and storing it as glycogen in the liver and muscles. Overnight, the body can use these stores of glucose, and both day and night, the liver calmly delivers just the right amount of glucose into the blood to provide energy for the rest of the body—every minute—whether you eat or not.

The graphs opposite show what happens.

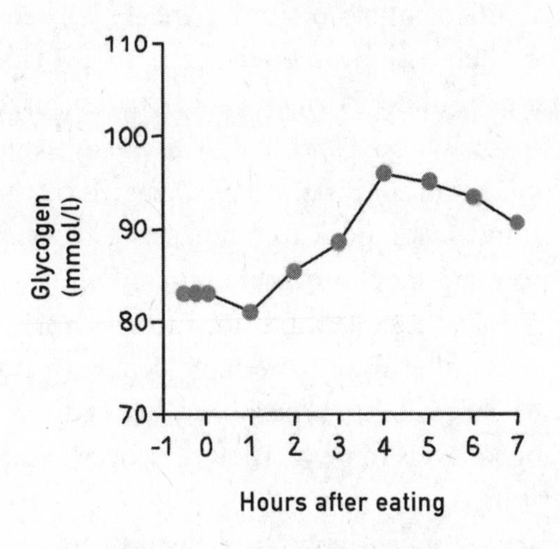

2.5a Change in muscle glycogen after eating breakfast only.

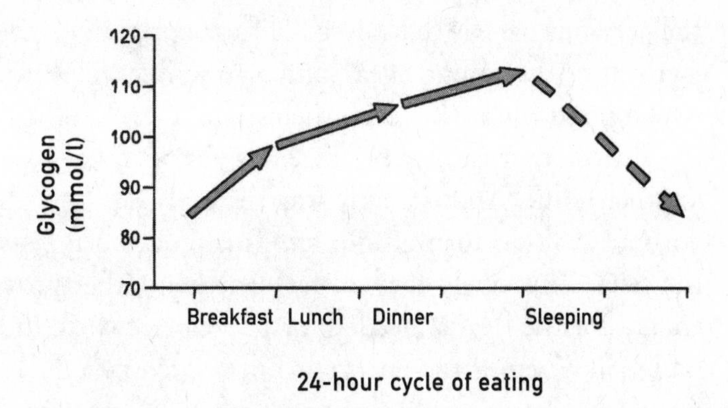

2.5b Increase in muscle glycogen during a day of eating 3 meals—and decrease during the night.

Once the tsunami of glucose from a meal has been tucked away, the fuel will be redistributed to provide energy for the rest of the body. Liver glycogen can be used to put glucose into the blood as needed. Muscle glycogen is broken down into short chains of carbon, carried by the blood to the liver and made back into glucose. Glycogen can also be used on the spot to power your muscle for a sudden burst of physical exertion, but for most sedentary people, it is just a useful temporary storage depot. In the graph, you can see that it takes around five hours after a meal for the glycogen levels to peak; then they decrease as the fuel is redistributed.

I say "temporary" storage depot, and that is certainly the ideal. But in Western society people typically eat three meals a day, leaving no time for the glycogen to be used. Instead, what happens as shown in the lower graph on the previous page is that there is a further rise in glycogen levels after the second meal, and again after the third, at which point the stores reach their highest level in the day.

Glucose that cannot be stored as glycogen has to find another home. And the only way the body has of dealing with it is to transform it into fat. This process happens in the liver. The newly formed fat can then either provide energy for the liver if needed, or be sent elsewhere in the body. However, if the energy is not needed in a 24-hour period, the levels stored there will gradually increase. Eat too much fat or carbohydrate, and fat will accumulate in the liver.

Overspill of Glucose Into Fat

The body can cope fine if you eat too much carbohydrate—in the short term. When the glycogen stores are full, the excess glucose has to be stored elsewhere. This is the key to understanding why surplus carbohydrate and fat share the same fate. Our bodies have only one way of handling this excess—it has to be transformed into fat.

That process—of transforming glucose into fat—happens only in the liver. But if this newly formed fat is not needed to burn for energy, then levels of fat stored in the liver will gradually increase. This process is of central importance for the development of type 2 diabetes, as will become clear.

Where Do You Store Your Fat?

It is no understatement to say that our ability to store energy as fat is the secret to our survival. If shipwrecked on a desert island, the average person can survive for many weeks without any food at all. First the body draws on glycogen—although this is a minor player as those stores will be exhausted after about 48 hours. Then, if there are still no ships on the horizon, it will turn to the fat stores. Body fat can provide us with all the energy we need for life for weeks.

The long string of carbon atoms that makes a fat molecule holds lots of energy. In every gram of fat, nine calories are locked up. A pound of fat contains just over 4,000 calories (or a kilogram 9,000 calories).

It is just the same for the fat in food, which is why fatty foods are also high-calorie foods. For fat in your body, the high-calorie content means efficient storage of energy.

Fat is stored mainly just under the skin. Some people are able to store lots of fat there, even though to our 21st-century eyes this may look undesirable. But for most of human history, it has been extremely desirable, signifying that they could afford to eat well and indicating a person's success and high social status. And there's another very potent factor that was recognized long ago: reproduction requires adequate nutrition, and undernourished people are less fertile. This is why images and artefacts symbolizing fertility all show very fat figures.

Humans tend to have a curious belief that if a little bit of something is good for you, then a lot is even better! Which is rarely true. Under the skin, fat is safely stashed away in a form that causes no harm to the rest of the body. However, although that comfy layer may not be a bad thing in itself, it may be an indicator that there could be too much elsewhere (see figures opposite and overleaf); and how much an individual can store in this safe, purpose-built storage layer varies a lot. If there is more fat than can be accommodated, the extra fat has to be stored elsewhere, such as within the stomach cavity. There it is known as "visceral" fat and is useful as a rough guide to how much excess fat the body has on board. The more visceral fat is present, the higher the risk of future heart attack—and diabetes.

Why? Well, because the presence of a lot of visceral fat,

although not *directly* dangerous, is an indication of something else that most definitely is, namely, fat accumulating inside the main organs—the liver, pancreas, heart, and muscle tissue. While the amount of visceral fat can be estimated with a tape measure around the waist, the fat that builds up inside the main organs is truly hidden. And, when it comes to the liver and pancreas, it can cause serious problems—of which more later.

In the next chapter, we shall see what conducts this whole orchestra of carbon moving around the body and why the music goes horribly wrong in type 2 diabetes.

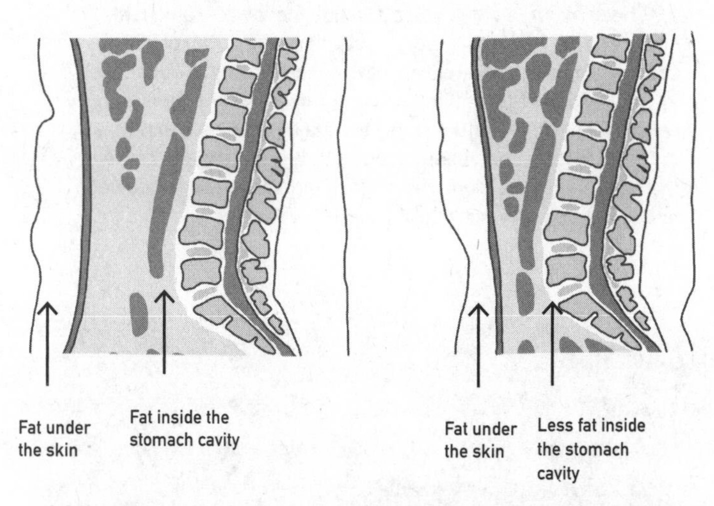

2.6 Looking at the body side on, these pictures show what is inside the lower trunk. The spine runs down the middle. Inside the tummy cavity, the loops of bowel show as gray and the rest is filled with the visceral fat (white). The left-hand scan picture shows a person with type 2 diabetes with a BMI of 35, and the right-hand picture shows the same person after losing 33 pounds in weight. The original MR scans can be viewed online at https://go.ncl.ac.uk/diabetes-reversal.

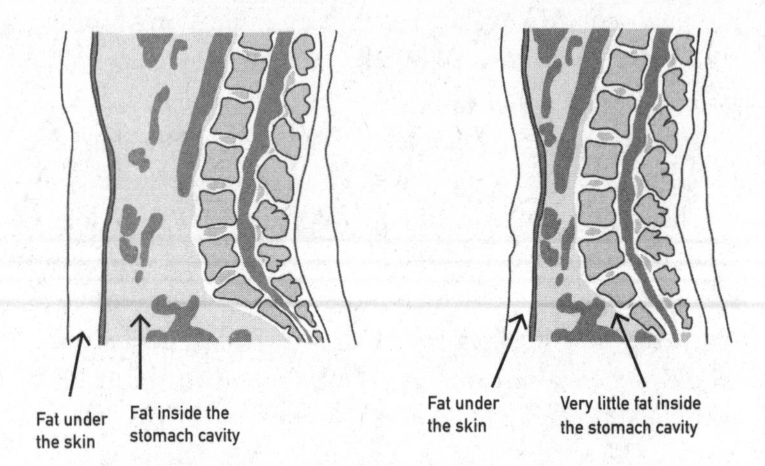

2.7 These pictures show what is inside the lower trunk, just like in Figure 2.6 but in a person starting with a BMI of 26. Once again, inside the tummy cavity, the loops of bowel show as gray and the rest is filled with the visceral fat (white). After weight loss (right-hand picture) the major change is that most of the visceral fat has been lost with only a modest decrease in the layer under the skin. The original MR scans can be viewed online at https://go.ncl.ac.uk/diabetes-reversal.

Quick Read

- The body spends most energy each day just on keeping itself alive
- Short periods of exercise burn relatively few calories and make little difference to the balance between calories eaten and calories used

- Long-duration physical activity—gardening, doing housework, walking around—can make a good contribution to long-term energy balance
- Humans get energy from only two basic types of fuel within the body—glucose and fat
- Glucose is stored as glycogen in the liver and muscle—but in small amounts
- Fat does not cause any metabolic problem when stored under the skin, but it can cause serious problems when it builds up in the main organs, especially the liver and pancreas

3

How Your Body Deals with Food

We are social animals. And a huge part of our social life centers on food: it oils the wheels of communication and is a framework for spending time with family and friends. This is all well and good—at least while we are young and healthy. The body deals with whatever is eaten—or drunk. We might eat to wild excess at a party, and take in far too much alcohol, but nothing too serious seems to result. Likewise, it copes if a meal is missed. The amazing body lives on.

But then, as adult life unfolds, our relationship with food tends to change. By now, food has become a habit. Rather than eating instinctively—and stopping when we have had enough—we eat because it's there and because we have got used to a certain amount of food, and we find it increasingly hard to skip a meal or change our routine. Nowadays, average adult body weight in the UK increases by a pound every year between the ages of 20 and 60. Some people gain only a little and some gain much more but the person who weighed 156 pounds at the age of 25 will on average weigh 176 pounds by the time they are 45. The upshot is that many people try to lose weight—often repeatedly. But the pressures of life—work, family, house, money—are relentless, and the main focus of life tends to be less on avoiding weight gain and more on dealing with whatever is most urgent. Sometimes, life just feels like survival. And throughout it all, the body lives on, seemingly oblivious to whatever is put into it—but getting heavier.

The way in which the body performs the miracle of keeping going whether you eat mainly cassava or mainly meat is astonishing.

Staying Alive Overnight

There is one organ that continues to demand the same amount of fuel throughout every 24-hour cycle. This organ is the brain. Day and night, your brain needs a steady and substantial amount of energy. It uses only one fuel—glucose—and, whether it is consciously busy or not, it uses the same amount. That may be disappointing news if at this moment you are tired after a long day of decision-making and planning. But the truth is that your brain will not have used more food-derived energy than if you had been daydreaming.

One funny thing about humans is that we have huge brains compared with other animals. You may well wonder how the brain gets enough fuel between meals, and especially overnight. Does it really depend upon glucose from the last meal? Surely not, given that blood glucose levels return to baseline just a few hours after eating and remain stable during the many hours spent asleep. So the glucose has to be coming from somewhere else.

Fortunately, a different organ has the very special job of keeping the glucose supply steady. This is the liver, as mentioned in Chapter 2. It keeps the brain supplied with glucose not just between meals but overnight too. The liver makes glucose every minute. In fact, most of the glucose in the blood comes not directly from food but from the liver.

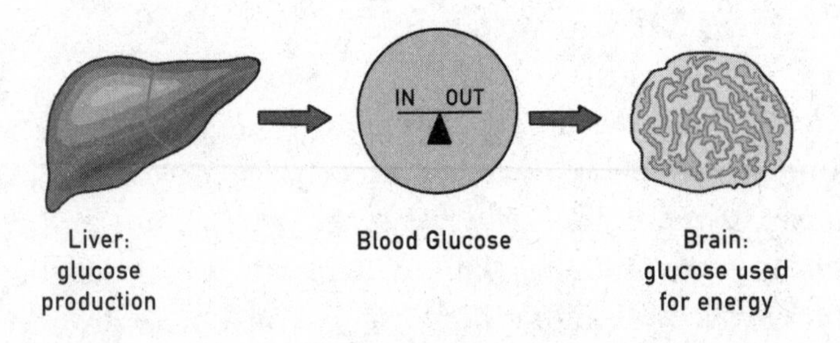

3.1 To keep the brain supplied with the glucose energy it must have, the liver makes glucose at just the right rate, and blood glucose levels stay steady.

Because the level of glucose in the blood is similar on going to bed and when waking up, it may seem as if nothing has happened. In fact, every morsel of glucose in the blood is changed every 90 minutes. As glucose is taken up and used by the brain, new glucose from the liver replaces it. It's just like a fast-flowing river, where the water is constantly moving on but the level remains constant.

During any period without food, the liver produces a constant, small amount of glucose for every two pounds of body weight. So, for instance, a man weighing 165 pounds would produce about one sixth of a gram every minute. In an hour, this adds up to about 10g of glucose (two teaspoonfuls). During your eight-hour sleep, eight times this amount, or about 80g (16 teaspoonfuls), is added to your blood. That is a lot of glucose to be made while your body is relatively inactive. To ingest the equivalent as carbohydrate, you would need to eat four thick slices of bread.

When you woke up this morning, every molecule of glucose in your blood had been manufactured by you, so they really were "sweet dreams." The brain demands, and the liver provides. All other tissues can rely on fat for energy.

This balancing act sounds quite simple—the liver puts the sugar into the blood for transport to the brain and the brain uses it to stay alive. But the link between usage and replacement is critical, and hidden. How does the liver know how much glucose to add to the blood?

The Role of Insulin

The answer is to be found in an amazing hormone called insulin. It really is the master controller of our internal "National Grid," regulating the supply of energy. Insulin is made in the beta cells, within the pancreas gland. It is the pancreas, hidden deep in the stomach cavity and quietly going about its business, that ensures that the right amount is released into the blood minute by minute. The plumbing for the pancreas is very clever, and different from other parts of the body. Blood passing through tissues is usually collected into veins, which take it back to the heart for general recirculation. But blood from the pancreas is collected into a special vein that delivers it straight to the liver.

Thus the insulin is not let loose into the whole body but immediately delivered to the liver, cutting out any delay in action. The fact that the system evolved in this way gives a clue to the most important action of insulin: it puts an immediate brake on the liver's enthusiasm to make more and more glucose. Left to its own devices, the liver would churn out large amounts of glucose.

What happens to control this is shown in the diagram opposite. If blood glucose starts to creep up, more insulin is made. If blood glucose starts to drop, less insulin is made. As insulin lasts only a few minutes in the blood, it achieves a very tight regulation of blood glucose by increasing or decreasing production according to requirements—with an immediate and direct impact on the liver.

What the Liver Sees

Your liver will respond to any increase in insulin levels by decreasing the amount of glucose released to the blood.

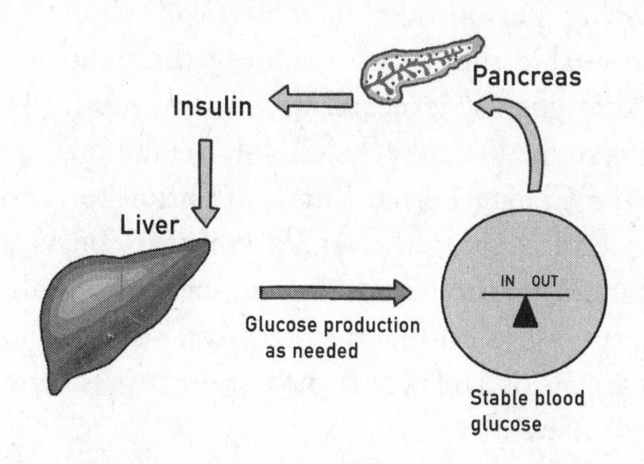

3.2 Normal control of glucose production by the liver—insulin restrains production to keep blood glucose stable and normal.

But the sensitivity of the liver to insulin varies from individual to individual. In 100 people, most will be nicely insulin-sensitive, some will be very sensitive, and some won't be sensitive at all. If a person's response is poor, we would describe their liver as "insulin-resistant." This phrase is bandied about a lot in explanations of type 2 diabetes—all too frequently as a mysterious harbinger of doom. The truth is much more interesting.

You might guess from the diagram above what happens if a liver is insulin-resistant. When the full effect of insulin is lacking, the liver makes more glucose than needed. As a result, blood glucose starts to creep up, and this causes more insulin to be made. Eventually, though, the liver gets the message, and blood glucose returns to normal.

Being insulin-resistant is not an inherently bad thing.

In a healthy person, the pancreas will simply work harder to enable the body to achieve the main goal—keeping that glucose level normal in the blood. It is an amazing system. As far back as 1854, the famous French physiologist Claude Bernard drew attention to the vital importance of keeping the *milieu intérieur* constant for all substances in the blood. An engineer may call it a feedback system—just like the thermostat in your house, which switches on the heat if the temperature drops and off when it rises.

One way of seeing whether a person is insulin-resistant is to measure the level of insulin in the blood first thing in the morning. Those people who are more insulin-resistant just run with higher insulin levels to keep control of their blood glucose.

The graph opposite shows the wide range of blood insulin levels in a large group of healthy people.

All organs in the body usually work at less than their maximum capacity. Your heart rate at rest might be around 70 beats per minute, although if you feel your pulse while climbing stairs it might be over 100 beats per minute. Yet your maximum heart rate could be as high as 180, depending on age and fitness. Also, you probably have two kidneys, but their job could be done by just half of one. The pancreas is the same. Normally, there is huge reserve capacity in the amount of insulin that can be made. We know that three quarters of the pancreas can be removed without blood glucose control being affected in most people. So compensating for an insulin-resistant liver is not usually a huge problem. The pancreas simply

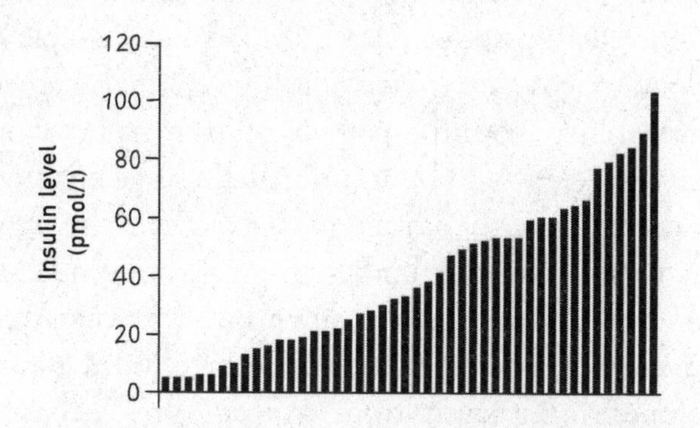

3.3 A wide range of insulin levels in 100 people without diabetes. Each bar shows the level in a group of healthy people.

works a little harder and, provided the insulin-producing cells can still compensate, blood glucose levels stay in the reasonable range. The people with the higher insulin levels shown in the graph above are normal, and all is still in balance.

But every pancreas has its limits, and when an insulin-resistant person builds up too much fat inside the pancreas, it may become unable to compensate fully, and that does become a problem, as we shall see later.

Quick, More Energy!

When your body is just ticking over at rest, fat can provide the energy for the muscles. But if you must catch that bus, the burst of muscle action can only be fueled by glucose. For instance, imagine your ancestors chasing after dinner with a spear. After no food for a couple of days, blood glucose levels would still be normal. If there was a sudden need to run—perhaps on hearing the shout of "Lion!"—there would be an immediate surge of adrenaline. Adrenaline is the hormone that triggers the fight-or-flight response in our bodies. It works very quickly, and one of its effects is to cut down insulin production. The liver starts to pour out more glucose, to provide more energy for sprinting away from danger—or for chasing dinner.

So the reason that you can live without thinking about energy for life is simple. Your liver organizes the fuel and produces exactly the right amount of glucose for the body. Your liver "knows" how much glucose to make, because insulin is in charge.

Surviving a Meal Onslaught

Taking on board a meal is a severe stress for the body. In the UK, a typical dinner of, say, 800 calories would probably contain around half of the energy as carbohydrate. That means 400 calories are eaten as carbohydrate, or the equivalent of 100g of carbohydrate. No matter how brown the rice, no matter how rustic the loaf, the body sees all food in a very prosaic manner. The digestible carbohydrate is converted into glucose (if you read the nutritional information on packets of food, carbohydrate is listed separately from sugar, but the process of digestion turns it all into sugar). Certainly, this happens more slowly with some forms of carbohydrate that are absorbed less rapidly. But your 800-calorie dinner, half made up of carbohydrate, will result in 100g of glucose being dropped into your body during digestion. This would cause disastrous effects unless rapid action occurred. In fact, if there was no insulin response, blood glucose would rise seven-fold. The normal level would go up to dangerous heights. You would feel very ill indeed.

Fortunately, rapid action is provided by the beta cells of the pancreas. When you start to eat your meal, blood glucose levels begin to rise. The moment that this happens, there is an enormous increase in the rate of insulin production. Blood levels of insulin increase 10–15 fold. Wow. That is the biggest change in any substance in the blood that can happen in normal adult life. If you imagine this in terms of speed, it is like accelerating from 10 miles per hour to over 100 miles per hour.

So what happens to all the extra insulin? Most of it goes directly to the liver. And within 30 minutes, production of glucose by the liver has almost completely stopped. Not just slowed, but almost stopped. The ongoing needs of your brain are supplied by glucose from food for a few hours.

The overall result is that in someone of normal health, blood glucose rises very little after a meal and the level returns close to normal within 90 minutes. A miracle. In the background, glucose is being steadily stored as glycogen in both the muscle and the liver.

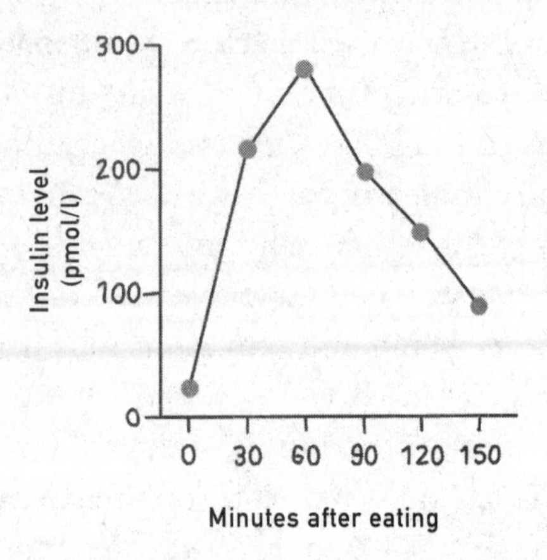

3.4 The normal insulin response to eating. Just after eating, the increase in blood insulin is startlingly rapid before falling again.

What Did You Do with Your Cornflakes?

Twenty-five years ago, I carried out some research in America that showed where you store away your meal carbohydrates. I had gone to work for a year at Yale University with my friend and colleague Jerry Shulman, after his team had discovered how to measure the level of glycogen in the body using special techniques on an MRI scanner. This was a game changer in terms of understanding what happens to the body after eating because for the first time its secrets could be probed without needles. Most carbon is non-magnetic, but exactly 1.1% of all carbon in nature is a slightly different form, known as carbon-13. And this, we now knew, could be measured using a very powerful MRI scanner. Changes in the level of carbon-13 exactly mirror changes in all carbon.

As a first step, we measured the levels of glycogen in a group of healthy people. There are only two storage depots for carbohydrates—the liver and the muscles—and we found that in these people about a third of the carbohydrate in a meal was stored in muscles and about a fifth in the liver. It took four to five hours after a meal for all the carbohydrate to be stored away (see figure 3.4).

This storage process is very dependent on insulin and, as we have seen, there is normally plenty around after a meal. But just as the liver's sensitivity to insulin can vary between individuals, so can muscle's. And what we found on continuing our research in the UK was that people with type 2 diabetes who had insulin-resistant muscles did not store anywhere near as much glycogen. Figure 3.5 on the next page shows just how big the difference was found to be.

So if you don't put much glucose into muscle, what happens to it? Well, as we saw in Chapter 2, some will be stored as glycogen in the liver. A small amount will certainly be burned for energy in the hours after a meal. But there is only one other option for the body to deal with the glucose influx. It has to be changed into fat. This is a neat solution, as there is much greater capacity to store fat.

Provided that it is burned for energy in a day or two, a temporary parking of extra carbohydrate in the form of fat does not matter too much. Into store it pops. Then out. No problem. The body remains in balance, day to day and

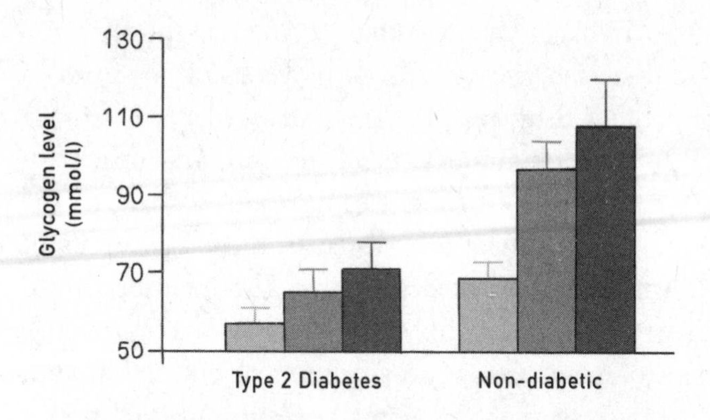

3.5 Amount of glucose stored as glycogen in muscles during a normal day. The lightest bars show the levels before breakfast. The dark gray bars show that the levels go up after breakfast, but by only a small amount in people with type 2 diabetes, compared with the large increase in storage in people without diabetes. The dark gray bars show that after lunch the muscle glycogen levels in type 2 diabetes have changed little from the fasting level whereas there was a large increase in those of people without type 2 diabetes.

week to week. But if, rather than the odd carbohydrate-heavy meal, you are eating a mouthful or two more food than you need *every day*, then that fat will slowly build up in the body and eventually in the liver too. Just how readily this happens depends on the degree of insulin resistance in your muscle, and this is why insulin resistance is not a good thing long term. The more insulin-resistant you are, the more likely you are to turn any excess carbohydrate into fat. The effects of this are explained in Chapter 4.

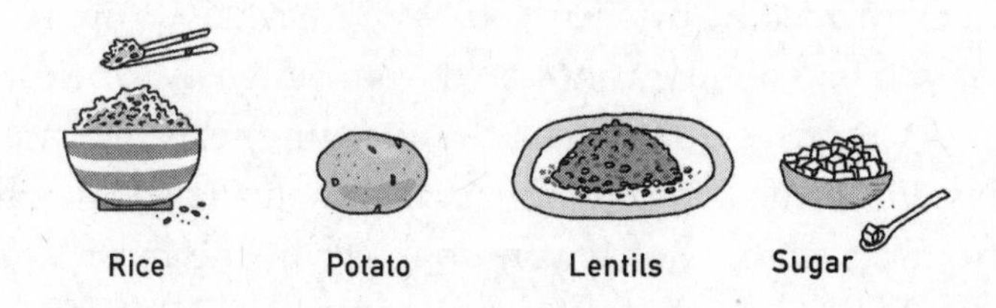

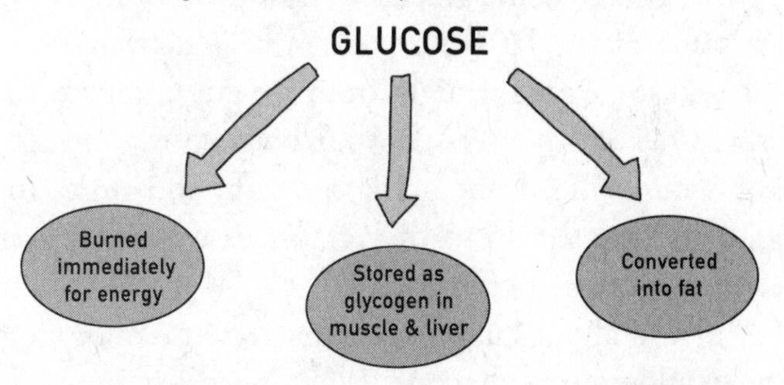

3.6 What happens to carbohydrate food once swallowed?

But What About the Fat in Our Food?

So far, we have talked mainly about the carbohydrates in our food and how they affect glucose levels; now it's time to look at what happens to the fat we eat. As you'll see in this section, the processing of fat and of glucose actually go hand in hand.

Let's return, briefly, to when you woke up this morning, and when your body was largely relying on fat for fuel. Fat was flowing from the fat stores to the tissues where it was required. Only the brain was burning glucose. That happy balance would have lasted until the first meal of the day. Ideally, by then you would have used up all the fat you had temporarily stored from yesterday's meals.

As soon as you eat in the morning, the increase in insulin in the blood rapidly switches off the release of fat from fat stores. But if you don't eat in the morning, or indeed for the rest of the day, your body will just continue to burn fat (and some glucose). After the first meal of the day, some of the fat from your meal is delivered to the liver, and some goes straight from the gut to muscle or fat tissue. Overall, this sets up your body so that all tissues have enough fuel to be going on with, and stores in fat tissues are topped up so they can release a steady supply between meals or overnight.

And how about surviving on that desert island? Exactly how would your body cope if marooned for weeks? Let's imagine that the essential water is available. But no food.

Different parts of the body have different requirements. We need to distinguish between the brain and the rest of the body here, because in normal life the brain can only burn glucose to keep going whereas the muscles and tissues can run on fat or glucose.

At first, in the absence of food, stores of glycogen in the liver and muscles will be used to provide the glucose that your brain demands. And during this time, everything will swing into action to minimize the use of glucose by the other muscles and tissues—which will gradually switch over to burning fat. After three days, however, the cupboard will be bare; glycogen stores will have been used up.

How does the brain survive without glucose being freely available? Never fear! Mammals have evolved another startling work-around. In the previous chapter, we saw that fat is made up of chains of carbon atoms. What this means is that, instead of burning the whole chain completely for energy, smart fuels can be made. These are ketones, and the brilliant thing is that these small molecules can easily diffuse into tissues. This includes brain cells, which adapt to the switch from glucose to ketones as fuel. The carbon links of the ketones are broken to release the essential energy, and the brain does just fine.

In fact, it can do very well indeed. Burning ketones seems to leave you alert and possibly less hungry. It enables you to focus without distraction on the matter of chasing after dinner. It is rumored that penniless artists, languishing in garret rooms, produce their best work from a ketone-powered brain. Some people find that their brain is at its sharpest in the early morning—hence epoch-changing discoveries being made before breakfast. Whether or not this is entirely the result of a ketone-fueled brain is still uncertain. What *is* certain is that ketones are the secret of our survival as a species despite famines and social upheavals.

If, for example, you had a long lie-in this morning, your ketone levels would be rising, and if you tested your urine, a small amount of ketones, normal for the circumstance, would be found. If you tested your urine immediately on being rescued from your desert island, you would find a moderately large amount of ketones, their presence merely indicating that your clever body is setting itself up to survive without much food coming in. It has devised a glucose substitute to power your brain.

You may have seen "ketogenic" diets advertised as "fat-burning" diets, but this rather distorts the truth. If less food is eaten than the body requires in any 24-hour period, then stored fat must indeed be burned, and this is so whatever the composition of the diet. There will be more ketones in urine than usual. If the diet is very low in carbohydrates, more of the calories will come from fat. Because the burning of fat from food will also yield ketones, the levels in the urine will be higher still—even though this is no guide to how much of your own body fat is being burned. Quite simply, weight loss will occur whenever less than the required calories are coming in from food. Cutting down on carbohydrates is successful in decreasing total calorie intake in some people, but there is no metabolic mystique to ketogenic diets.

Why Your Doctor Fears Ketones

There is a dark side to ketones. Doctors and nurses tend to fear them, and this is for one reason. In type 1 diabetes—a very different disease from type 2—the body is completely dependent upon insulin being injected. If insulin is not injected for any reason or if illness demands a much higher insulin dose, the severe insulin deficiency causes the liver to produce a huge amount of ketones. This can lead to a life-threatening condition—known as diabetic ketoacidosis—for which urgent lifesaving treatment is needed.

There is usually no doubt if ketones are worryingly high—i.e., far, far above the levels seen during normal fasting—but ordinary levels of ketones are broadly good: they are the molecules of survival.

The Secret Life of the Pancreas

So far in this chapter we have considered the normal regulation of metabolism in health. Control by insulin is central to the whole business so we should consider in more detail the organ that produces it and calls the shots in health (and in type 2 diabetes).

The pancreas is a shy organ. It hides away and does its vital job of making insulin without fuss—normally. It controls what you do with food and how you provide energy for everything. Insulin is known as the master regulator of metabolism because it is by far the most powerful controller of your energy supply. Other hormones have modest effects on what happens to glucose, but insulin can override these.

Where is your pancreas? Few people know, although they know perfectly well where their heart, their brain, or their liver can be found. The pancreas lies at the back of the stomach cavity, partly behind and partly below the stomach itself. This is shown in figures 3.7 and 3.8. Put your hand over the front lower edge of your ribs on your left side—then it will be over your stomach. Your pancreas is deep inside, below your hand. In comparison, other organs are easy to study. Brain specialists have a neatly packaged organ to focus upon. Liver specialists have a big lump of an organ to scan or sample with needles, and heart specialists have a dinky little pump that is very accessible for insertion of tubes or for scans.

In contrast, the pancreas is difficult. It is an irregular,

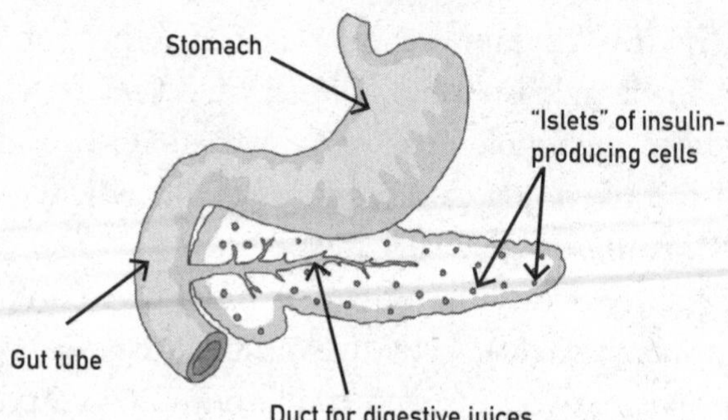

3.7 The pancreas has "islets" of insulin-producing cells scattered throughout. Its other job is to make digestive juices and deliver these to the gut tube.

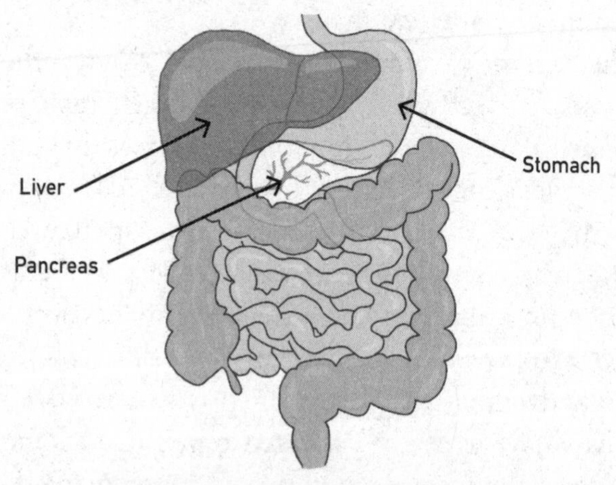

3.8 This is where the pancreas lives. The picture shows what would be seen when looking straight at a person's body but with the "lid" removed. The duct of the pancreas can be seen running down its middle. The long tail of the pancreas disappears from view behind the stomach.

floppy organ whose broad end sits hard up against the first few inches (10cm) of the small intestine and then tapers gradually to a tip far over on your left-hand side, bending up and over your spinal column. Overall, it is very hard to get in focus—on a scan for instance—because it lurks at the very back of the stomach cavity, behind the spleen, and embedded in a layer of fat. A cynic might say that the pancreas was designed as a joke on diabetes specialists!

As a result, the pancreas is the least studied organ in diabetes. Which is astonishing, given that it is the most important.

And then, to top it all, the pancreas is not one organ, but two. Part deals with digestion of food, and part makes hormones.

Most of the pancreas's bulk is devoted to making the digestive juices that flow into the gut to break down food into what the body wants. It is made up of tiny lobules that busily make the juices, each lobule having a tiny drainage duct. The tiny lobules are grouped together into irregularly shaped larger lobules from which small drainage tubes flow into a main tube running the length of the pancreas and delivering the juices to the intestine. These larger lobules are separated by sheets of fatty tissue. But none of this is directly related to making insulin.

Of the various hormones in our bodies, only a handful are vital. Along with insulin, these include thyroxine, cortisol, estrogen, and testosterone, each of which is made by a special, distinct organ: the thyroid gland in the neck, the adrenal gland above each kidney, and the ovaries or testes respectively. Nothing so simple for our friend insulin, however! For insulin is made not by a single, identifiable organ, but by clusters of cells called beta cells, which are scattered throughout the pancreas gland. And because, under the microscope, these clusters look like little islands in a sea of other tissue, they are known as "islets."

Until recently, all that we knew about the human pancreas came from looking at the dissected organ after death or after surgical removal because of disease. The lack of study was partly because of its awkward position in the body and its shape. But now, thanks to special MR studies, we know more about it than ever before. These special studies led to the findings that underpin this book. They have enabled us not just to gain full view of the pancreas but to measure the level of fat within it.

How Big Is Your Pancreas?

One day in 2014, clutching a pair of images, one of my team at our research center in Newcastle burst excitedly into my office. Dr. Mavin Macauley had spent two years measuring the size of the pancreas in people with type 2 diabetes. It had been a struggle. But now he had started to measure the pancreas in people without diabetes, and he just could not believe his eyes. There it was, obvious at a glance. Compared with the small, ragged pancreases of people with type 2 diabetes that Mavin had tussled with for so long (and had assumed were normal in size and shape), here was one of princely size—and then another lovely plump one.

Eureka moments in science are rare but to be enjoyed! It is often said that medical research is 99% perspiration and 1% inspiration, but we could add that it's also 99.9% slog and 0.1% huge excitement. Figure 3.9 shows pancreases from two people of the same sex of a similar age and weight, but only one has type 2 diabetes. These images show just what Mavin was so excited about. It does not take an expert to see the difference.

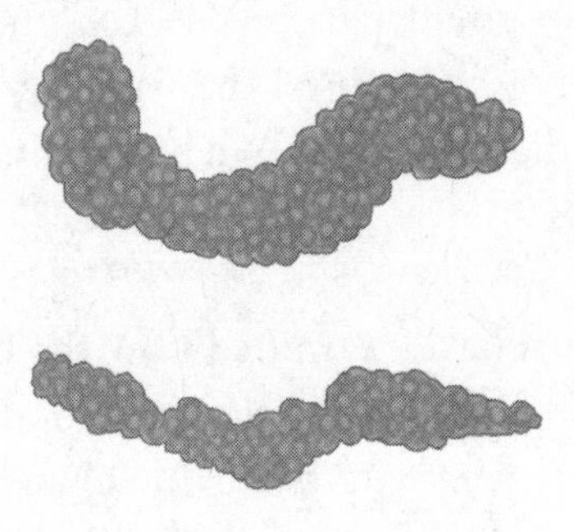

3.9 3-D images of the human pancreas derived from MRI scans. The pancreas at the top is from a person with normal glucose control and the one at the bottom is from a person with type 2 diabetes.

The discovery that the pancreas of people with type 2 diabetes was only about two thirds of the size of the pancreas of non-diabetic people of the same sex and similar age and weight sent us scurrying to the library to find out if other scientists had noticed this. A few had indeed, but because such a vast number of scientific papers are published every year, sometimes important information is available but not widely noted. If scientists pick up new concepts en route and write them into summary articles, these *may* become widely discussed and eventually incorporated into textbooks. But, at the time of writing this book, very few diabetes specialists know that a person with type 2 diabetes has a shrunken pancreas.

What did it mean that the pancreas was smaller in type 2 diabetes? There were two possibilities. Maybe, we surmised, people who were more prone to type 2 diabetes had been born with rather small pancreases. On the other hand, perhaps something had caused the pancreas to shrink as a consequence of diabetes itself? We had to find out.

In this chapter we have examined how the body works in normal life, i.e., before the development of diabetes, when the pancreas just keeps its head down and ensures that your food is stored or used for energy in the optimum way. In the next, we will look at what happens when the pancreas can't do its job anymore—and why.

Quick Read

- Life revolves around supplying the brain with glucose

- This constant supply comes mainly from the liver
- Insulin regulates the release of glucose from the liver to keep blood glucose constant
- Insulin also controls where meal carbohydrate is stored
- People vary in how sensitive their muscles are to insulin
- Insulin resistance in muscle leads to the conversion of glucose to fat
- During food shortage, ketones are made to compensate for the lack of glucose

4

Type 2 Diabetes: A Bad Case of Food Poisoning

Even water can be bad for you—in large quantities. Simply by drinking far too much you may die. Water intoxication is a real thing. Although we may think of a poison as a substance that is inherently toxic, in reality it is often the dose of the substance that dictates the harm. For instance, vitamins are essential for life, but some can be toxic if too large a quantity is taken. Alcohol can enhance enjoyment of life in small doses, but it can lead to serious illness and death in excess.

In just the same way, food can enhance enjoyment of life. But, sadly, if you take even a little more than your body needs over a long period of time, you will run into problems. For those who are susceptible, the most hazardous of these problems is type 2 diabetes. Most people can deal with excess amounts of food without getting diabetes. The arbitrary cut-off that defines "obesity" has nothing to do with type 2 diabetes: you do not have to be obese to develop the condition. You simply have to be susceptible to excess fat . . . in the wrong place. That is the key to understanding why the insidious long-term poison of excess food might or might not bring about diabetes.

The term "food poisoning" has traditionally been used to describe acute upsets. But perhaps it is now appropriate to broaden its use, to draw attention to the chronic problems in our society today caused by the constant availability of food.

If you have type 2 diabetes, your body will have had more food than it needed to burn over many years. Your fat stores will be full to the brim. In fact, your body will be drowning in excess chemical energy. And when fuel tanks overspill, there are inevitably serious consequences. This chapter describes what is going on in your body if you have developed type 2 diabetes, and why it developed in the first place.

Changes as a Result of Type 2 Diabetes

Your Blood

The obvious thing is that your blood glucose levels are too high. That bit is easy. Blood glucose levels can be measured using one of the widely available meters. The glucose itself might cause you to be thirsty and pass more urine than usual.

Less well known is the fact that the levels of insulin in your blood will be higher than normal. That may surprise you. It certainly confuses medical students! It is the result of your pancreas trying as hard as possible to restore glucose levels to normal. Then, eventually, after many years of type 2 diabetes, insulin levels gradually decline because the poor old beta cells become less and less able to do their job.

The levels of ordinary fat in your blood will also be too high. This is because some of the excess glucose in your blood will be transformed into fat—fat that should be stashed away in the fat stores under the skin, except that they are already full to the brim.

Given that glucose, insulin, and fat have vital roles to play in keeping you alive, it is fair to describe the whole picture as metabolic mayhem. No wonder you may not feel at your best.

The graphs below show how blood levels of glucose, insulin, and fat compare between people with type 2 diabetes and similar people without diabetes. The average levels over 24 hours are shown.

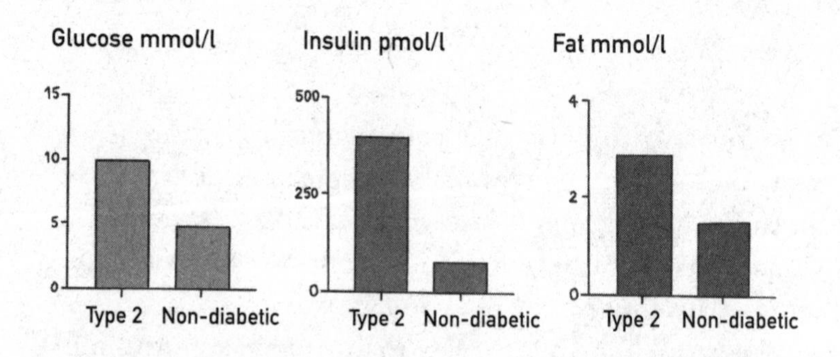

4.1 Average levels over 24 hours for blood glucose, insulin, and fat, in people with type 2 diabetes compared with people without diabetes.

Your Pancreas

As mentioned in Chapter 1, type 2 diabetes only develops if the beta cells in the pancreas have become unable to respond normally to glucose. It had long been believed by medical researchers that these cells were dying off gradually, one by one. Why? Looking at a postmortem pancreas under the microscope, scientists could see that there were about half the normal number of insulin-producing cells. Most scientists and doctors believed that there were different causes for this in different people. Yet in type 2 diabetes, a single factor stands out. The condition is rare in populations short of food but common in those with plenty of food. And, if populations with plenty of food suddenly run into food rationing, type 2 diabetes becomes far less common, as was documented in Cuba after the economic collapse in the 1990s. Such a simple change determining the frequency of a disease implies one single cause.

Overnight, in a person with type 2, the remaining beta cells try to control blood glucose levels but it's a struggle. Then, after eating, the problem becomes very clear. The beta cells can walk, gradually managing to pump more insulin into the blood, but they cannot run in response to a sudden demand. Try as they might, the beta cells have become incapable of responding rapidly to rising blood glucose levels. The demand for a surge in insulin production goes unanswered. That is really the hallmark of type 2 diabetes—lack of a rapid response to demand.

Your Liver

If you have type 2 diabetes, your liver will be insulin-resistant. As explained in Chapter 3, this lack of response to the controlling hormone, insulin, will make it unable to shut off the production of glucose. Consequently, glucose pours into the blood.

This happens not only throughout the night but also during the day. It continues after you eat your breakfast. So instead of glucose production stopping to make room for the incoming flood of glucose from meal carbohydrates, your body has to deal with a double whammy. Food is causing the glucose level to rise but your liver is cheerfully shoveling more into the blood at the same time.

One other job of your liver after meals is to store glucose as glycogen. You will be relieved to know that your liver does this just fine, even with your type 2 diabetes. This is because the liver gets the hint that it needs to make glycogen whenever the blood glucose level rises. Liver cells have no barrier to glucose so it floods into them, and is then turned into glycogen. That is okay, but the liver can store only a relatively small amount of glucose as glycogen.

Your Muscle

The earliest detectable clue that someone is likely to develop type 2 diabetes in the future is that their muscles are relatively resistant to insulin. That is to say, insulin, the master controller of the metabolism, cannot fully switch on the uptake of glucose in muscle. This will have been true from childhood. It is mainly determined by the mixture of genes you happen to inherit. The lack of a full response to insulin does not cause any immediate problems and most people are unaware of it. Their muscle will simply be more insulin-resistant than that of their friends who are not destined to develop type 2 diabetes.

Chapter 3 describes what happens to the carbohydrate in meals, in a person with normal sensitivity to insulin in their muscle: after breakfast, the rise in blood insulin levels causes the muscles in the body to start taking up much more glucose and storing it as glycogen. The muscle stores do a very important job in allowing safe storage of glucose to cope with the huge influx from each meal. That food energy is later passed on to other tissues. Muscle normally acts as a dynamic buffer, smoothing out the swings in blood glucose that would otherwise happen. As all the muscle together make it the largest organ in the body, this is important.

But in those prone to type 2 diabetes, storage of glucose as glycogen in muscle is inadequate. The pie charts below show the results of one of our very early studies applying magnetic resonance to try to understand type 2 diabetes. This study involved measuring the amount of glycogen in thigh muscle before, and then at intervals after, breakfast then lunch. The chart in figure 4.2 shows the increase in glycogen stores in people who do not have muscle insulin resistance. But just look at what happens to the people who do. They are unable to store more than a tiny fraction of the meal carbohydrate as muscle glycogen.

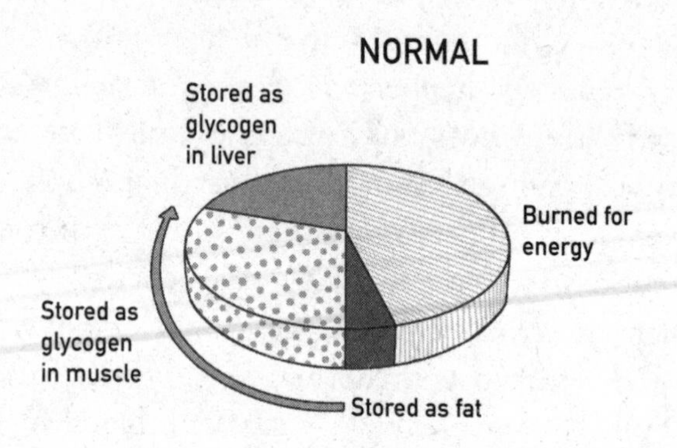

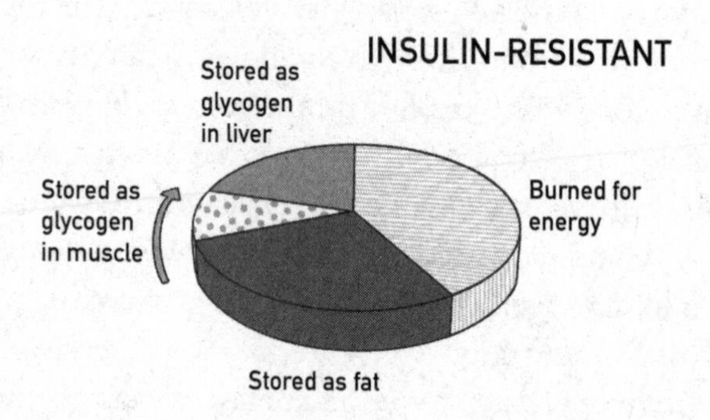

4.2 Where do you store your meal carbohydrate? Normally around one third is stored in muscle (upper panel). But if the muscles are insulin-resistant then much less can be stored and the rest is turned into fat (lower panel).

If the glucose is refused entry into muscle it has to stay in the blood. No wonder blood glucose shoots up after breakfast and usually stays high all day. But something has to be done, and as we know from Chapter 3, the only other way the body has of dealing with excess glucose is to turn it into fat. As the pie charts show, in people with insulin-sensitive muscles, only a minute proportion of the carbohydrate in a meal is turned into fat, but in people with insulin-resistant muscle, this rises to around a quarter.

Being forced to make fat may seem a rather gloomy fate—particularly as you are stuck with the genes that determine your general level of muscle insulin resistance. But there is a clear message here: if a person keeps their weight healthy throughout adult life, there is no excess fuel hanging around from day to day. Anything initially changed into fat will be used in that 24-hour period, tiding the body over to the following day. On the other hand, if not all the fat is used, it will slowly silt up in the body. Remember: no excess food, no food poisoning.

There is another vital message: insulin resistance in muscle can be moderately improved by exercise. Over many years, this will have a considerable effect on health. Regular exercise is a great way to delay or prevent the onset of type 2 diabetes, although once the damage has been done it is usually too little too late. The younger you are when you start, the greater the benefit over a lifetime. You will share many of your genes with family members. So if you have type 2 diabetes, it is even more important that you set an example for your children, nieces, nephews, or grandchildren. Get them in the habit of walking whenever possible, as well as cycling and playing outside.

When Did Things Start to Go Wrong?

You may wonder when things started going out of kilter and your type 2 diabetes began to develop. Just a few months ago? Last year?

A remarkable study that followed people over a very long time was able to throw some light on the years leading up to the onset of type 2 diabetes. This was the Whitehall 2 study. It involved repeated blood tests on 6,538 civil servants, and observed what happened over time. Eventually, of course, some people developed type 2 diabetes. In fact, over 500 people—around 1 in 10—did so. And, because blood samples had been taken and stored every year, it was possible to find out how fast the blood glucose went up before the diabetes was diagnosed.

Even 13 years before diagnosis, blood glucose was raised—just a tiny bit. It then gradually increased so that over almost a decade the average blood glucose had risen from 5.5 to 5.8mmol/l. This was still well within the normal range (of up to 6.1mmol/l). But then, especially in the 18 months before diagnosis of type 2 diabetes, things started moving more rapidly, with a sharp rise in blood glucose to an average of 7.4mmol/l by the time the condition was confirmed. This is shown in the graph in figure 4.3.

Keep in mind that this information is based on average data from a large group and reflects the average person's path to type 2 diabetes. Your own path may be different. For example, if you put on a moderate amount of weight

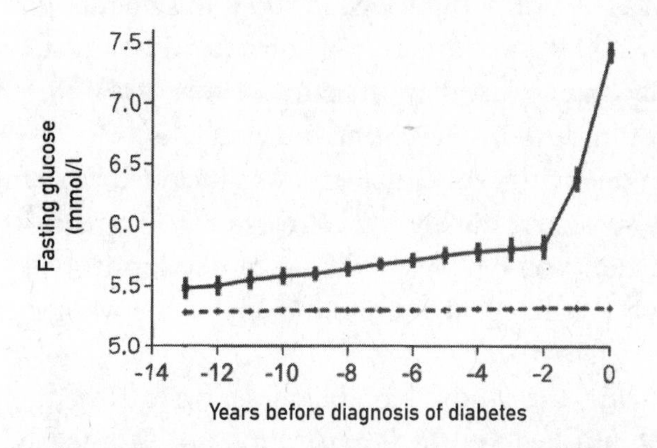

4.3 Blood glucose before breakfast rises very slowly—it is usually over a decade before diabetes appears (solid line). There is then a relatively rapid rise in the couple of years leading up to diabetes appearing. People who do not develop type 2 diabetes keep steady, normal glucose levels (dotted line).

in your 20s and 30s, then remained at a steady weight, type 2 diabetes coming on at age 60 may have been percolating away gently for 30 years. If, on the other hand, you had remained at a steady weight between the ages of 20 and 55, then had piled on the weight, it is possible that your diabetes, also diagnosed at the age of 60, may have been rumbling for only four or five years. Remember that averages are only useful on average.

WOSCPS

As acronyms go, WOSCPS is one of the most memorable. It stands for "The West of Scotland Coronary Prevention

Study." This study, published in 1995, was not designed to provide clues about how type 2 diabetes developed, but it managed to do just that. (Its purpose was to test the effect of a statin drug in preventing heart attacks.)

No one with type 2 diabetes was included at the start of the study but during the course of the five years it was conducted, some people went on to develop it. It is very common. It happened to around 1% of the whole group over the five years.

During the study, blood samples were stored. After it had finished, my colleague Professor Naveed Sattar in Glasgow had the brilliant idea that these six-monthly blood samples could be put to good use. No one knew what detailed changes in the blood happened in the years leading up to type 2 diabetes. And what Professor Sattar realized was that, because at the end of the study the participants could be divided into two groups—those who had developed type 2 diabetes and for comparison those who had not—the stored blood samples could show how the body had been changing *before* type 2 diabetes was diagnosed. This information was published in 2008 and helped formulate my Twin Cycle Hypothesis, of which more in the next chapter.

The graphs show the results of two important blood tests over the 18 months before diagnosis. First, levels of fat in the blood were abnormally high in those on track to develop type 2 diabetes (almost 50% higher). Second, the ALT test, which is the best indicator of distress in the liver, was raised compared with levels in those who did not develop diabetes.

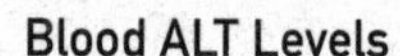

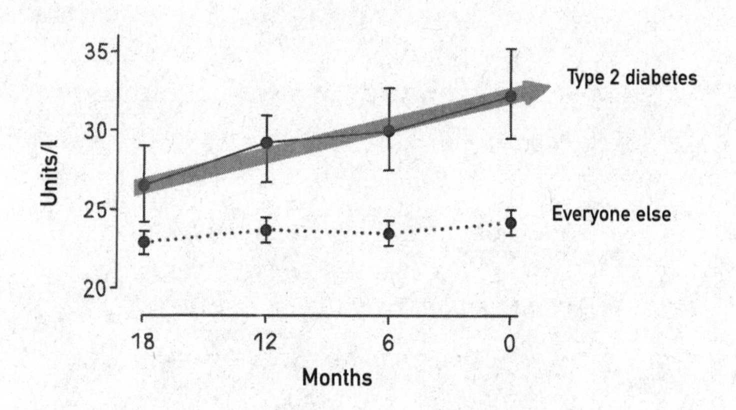

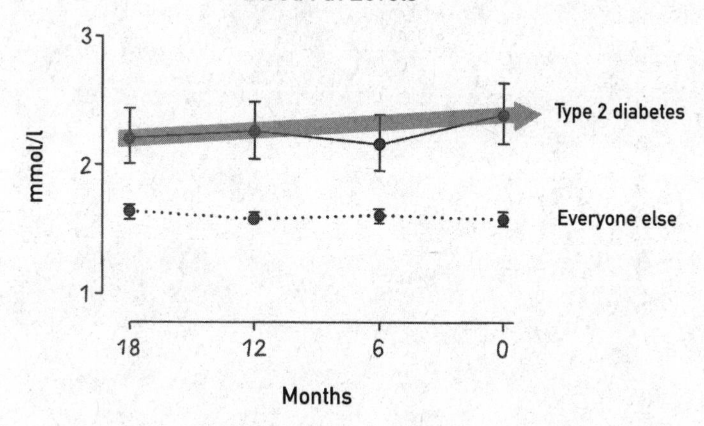

4.4 Changes in the blood before type 2 diabetes appears. The gray arrows indicate the overall trends. The top graph shows that the ALT test is already raised 18 months before diagnosis, and is rising rapidly—indicating a stressed liver. The bottom graph shows that the level of fat in the blood must have become abnormal even before the study began.

So even though they did not know it, as they hurtled down the path to diabetes, their livers were giving out a long, silent scream.

Quick Read

- Food is essential for life, but can be toxic if too much is consumed over a long period of time
- In type 2 diabetes, the pancreas cannot make enough insulin at the right time
- In addition, the liver and muscles do not respond normally to whatever insulin is around
- As a result, the liver makes too much glucose
- At the same time, the muscles cannot store glucose after meals
- Result: too much glucose in the blood

5

A Murder Mystery and the Twin Cycles

Who Dunnit?

There had been disappearances and murder was suspected. The victims were the beta cells. When pancreas tissue from people with type 2 diabetes was looked at under a microscope, it seemed that half of the beta cells had simply disappeared. Missing, presumed dead. And in people whose diabetes had been long-standing, almost two thirds of the cells had gone. It appeared conclusive that the beta cells were being murdered, one by one. What was going on? Could the killer be brought to justice?

In 2006, as described in the introduction, I came face-to-face with that graph showing that the high blood glucose levels in type 2 diabetes could be normalized in seven days. The scientific paper that reported this was about bariatric surgery, carried out to bring about weight loss in very heavy people. The authors suggested that the rapid change in blood glucose might be due to hormones made by the gut—the incretin hormones. It was 35 years since

I had listened as a medical student to Professor Reginald Passmore predicting the existence of these hormones, and they had subsequently been identified. It was pleasing to see just how correct his scientific deduction had been. But these incretin hormones were extremely unlikely to be the reason why early-morning blood glucose levels had so rapidly changed, as described in the paper. Incretin hormones simply could not do that. They do not have a major effect on blood glucose overnight and in the early morning; they work almost entirely after meals. And we knew that those people undergoing stomach surgery had not eaten anything in the seven days since the operation. No meals—no increase in incretin hormones. All of this was a valuable insight. Because if the incretin hormones were not causing the glucose to change then something else was.

Details of the Case

In type 2 diabetes, half the beta cells seemed to have been murdered. Who were the suspects? From the Passmore insights, Mr. Incretin seemed to have an alibi. Other popular villains included the mysterious Ms. Amyloid and Mr. Inflammation.

Amyloid is a substance that is sometimes observed in the islets of people with type 2 diabetes. Belief in amyloid as a cause of beta cell death in type 2 diabetes became quite widely established in the 1980s, but on the flimsiest of evidence. It has lurked as a potential villain since, but although Ms. Amyloid might have the means on theoretical grounds, she is only occasionally present at the scene of the crime.

Inflammation can cause lots of problems in many different parts of the body. It can sometimes be a killer—for instance, in childhood or type 1 diabetes. In that very different type of diabetes, an immune attack by inflammatory cells is absolutely central to the problem of beta cell death. But in type 2 diabetes, the extent of inflammation seemed insufficient to be threatening as a murder weapon. So Mr. Inflammation was not high on the suspect list, either by means or by presence at the scene.

Let's take a hint from all the great detectives of fiction. We should pause and reassess the crime. How about this business of the apparent recovery of the beta cell after seven days? Was the fall in blood glucose anything to do with the beta cell itself? After all, type 2 diabetes comes on over many years, and sudden resurrection does not happen at a murder scene. What was going on?

Step forward, Mr. Liver. Research in Newcastle and elsewhere had shown how the liver controls blood sugar at all times. It controls the flow of glucose both during the night and after eating—rather poorly in people with type 2 diabetes. And we know that the liver sets the blood glucose level in response to insulin. Over the eight years leading up to that important day in 2006, we had been researching the effect of fat inside the liver and had discovered that excess fat was potent in preventing insulin from doing its job. The fat itself was making the liver insulin-resistant.

My close colleagues at Yale University in the U.S., Kitt Petersen and Jerry Shulman, had shown just the previous year that moderate food restriction over a couple of months could improve liver fat levels. And that this in turn improved the response of the liver to insulin. I worked with Jerry and Kitt, living beside Long Island Sound in 1990–91, and knew how carefully they conducted scientific studies. Their work, my work, and all previous observations on liver fat suddenly clicked together to explain the dramatic normalization of blood sugar only seven days after bariatric surgery. It also explained what might be happening to the beta cells.

Deduction

It went like this: the people in the bariatric surgery study were of course very heavy. That is why they were having the operation. It was simple to work out approximately how many calories they would need every 24 hours just to stay alive. They would require at least 2,700 calories every day, just lying in bed all day, not moving a muscle. That is more than the average person eats even when they are moving around. Before a surgeon operates on the stomach, of course, no eating is allowed for at least 12 hours. The usual food intake for these people had suddenly dropped, from a very considerable amount to zero on the evening before surgery, when the nurse hung a sign on their bed: "nil by mouth." The body must stay alive—and would still need 2,700 calories to do so every day. Over the seven days following the operation, seven times this amount would need to be found—a total of 19,000 calories. A small number would be provided by supporting fluids given into a vein, but the vast majority would have to be found elsewhere.

Fortunately for all of us, our bodies are built for survival, with stores for a rainy day. And just look at that available fuel, sitting there in the liver poised for action. The heavier a person, the more likely they are to have large amounts of fat inside the liver. We knew that this particular store of fat is used first. It is far easier for the body to mobilize energy from the central organ of metabolism than to retrieve fat from the long-term storage depot under the skin. So it seemed likely that in those bariatric patients the liver fat levels might have dropped rapidly. Supposing that had caused the insulin resistance of the liver to decrease equally rapidly? In turn, the sudden return of a normal response to insulin would surely switch off the previous outpouring of glucose. Very suddenly. According to this reasoning, the rapid change in blood glucose could be a simple consequence of using up excess liver fat and nothing to do with the beta cell.

So maybe the rapid normalization of blood glucose was not due to the surgeon's undoubted and fantastic skill but just reflected that sign hanging on the bed—nil by mouth? Of course, people can eat again a week or so after undergoing that particular type of surgery, but their stomachs will have been cut down to a fraction of the original size (to approximately the size of your thumb). They continue to be very limited regarding how much food they can consume. Therefore the sudden improvement in blood glucose would surely be maintained.

But what about the presumed murder scene? What about the beta cells? Surely the change in blood glucose at seven days was nothing to do with them? They could not be expected to recover magically in a week, whoever the villain turned out to be.

Remember that type 2 diabetes behaves in populations as though there was a single cause. What if—just what if—the drop in liver fat was mirrored by a drop in fat content of the pancreas? Could this allow normal function of the pancreas to return, in such a way that insulin could be made normally again? If it was all due to excess fat, as in the liver, then there might indeed be one simple cause for type 2 diabetes, not separate causes in different organs, as had been believed.

Visions of liver, fat, beta cell, and life appeared in a glorious melange, changing places with each other. All the right ideas were there, but, to borrow a phrase from Eric Morecambe, not necessarily in the right order. One of the most important sets of scientific equipment is the least expensive: a blank sheet of paper, a pencil, and the human brain. Each detail could be written down, considered in relation to other items, rubbed out, and moved. *Had* there been a murder? What actually caused what? Which came first? How are they all connected? It took several months to capture the ideas in a diagram.

Ladies and gentlemen, there had been no murder. The beta cells were surely still alive—even though "disappeared."

The Twin Cycles

First, the Liver Cycle

On that sheet of paper, the ideas gradually settled into a pattern that reflected what we knew. There had to be two vicious cycles that interacted. The first one happened in the liver. By taking a mouthful or two more food each day than your body actually needs, you very gradually increase your liver fat levels. This is exacerbated by the fact that, because your muscles have been relatively insulin-resistant from birth, they do not store the normal amount of glucose after each meal. Instead, the glucose is taken up by the liver and turned into fat. The gradually increasing insulin resistance causes the liver to make more glucose and your poor beleaguered pancreas to make a little more insulin.

But it is a fact of life that insulin actually *speeds up* the conversion of glucose to fat in the liver . . . and so the whole unfortunate cycle begins again, causing the level of liver fat to go up further, with all the unfortunate knock-on effects.

Figure 5.1 shows how these events are linked.

Having too much fat inside it, your liver very reasonably tries to shunt it off to safe storage in the layer under

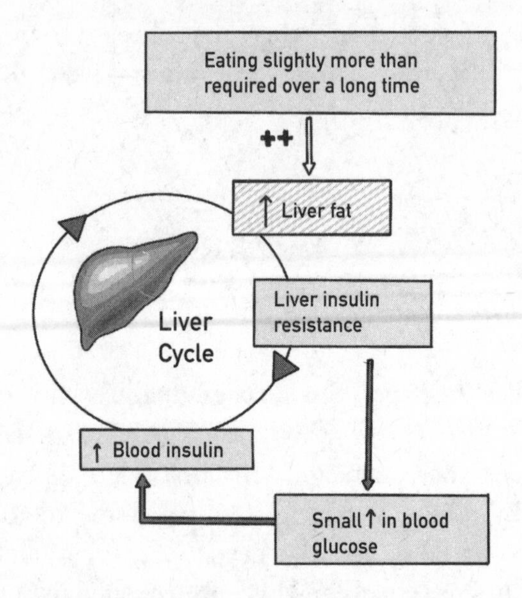

5.1 Twin cycle hypothesis: First of the twin cycles—the vicious cycle in the liver. An extra mouthful of food daily over a long period of time causes fat in the liver to build up. This makes the liver unable to respond properly to insulin. Blood glucose starts to creep up and this causes higher background levels of insulin. This insulin then oils the wheels for glucose to be turned into liver fat.

the skin, increasing the rate at which it exports fat into the blood. Some people have almost unlimited safe storage capacity for fat, and if so, diabetes may not happen for a long time. But in some people this depot under the skin is already full, and so the level of fat in their blood stays too high.

Have you ever had a full cupboard, been forced to put things elsewhere and then been annoyed by them being left in inconvenient places? Imagine the rest of your body being exposed to long-term high levels of fat in the blood. Eventually, the fat is going to build up in inconvenient places. One such place might be inside the pancreas.

Then, the Pancreas Cycle

Back to that piece of paper. Assuming that the presence of fat in the pancreas did gum up the works and prevent insulin from being made rapidly after meals, we could expect a gradual blunting of the normal insulin response to eating, which in turn would lead to raised blood glucose levels for longer after meals. It was already known that in people with type 2, the mealtime response of insulin becomes inadequate before the condition comes on. But now I could see that the prolonged high glucose levels would also cause a rise in the background level of insulin in the blood, and that in the liver this would also cause a further rise in the conversion of glucose into fat.

Once established, these two vicious cycles will interact and reinforce each other. Too much fat from the liver will drive the pancreas cycle, and high glucose levels will eventually force up the insulin levels, driving the liver cycle.

In 2007, I presented these tentative answers as a lecture to the annual UK Diabetes Conference in Glasgow. Fortuitously, the editor of the main European diabetes journal was in the audience and asked me to write up the hypothesis as a paper for publication. That was a challenge.

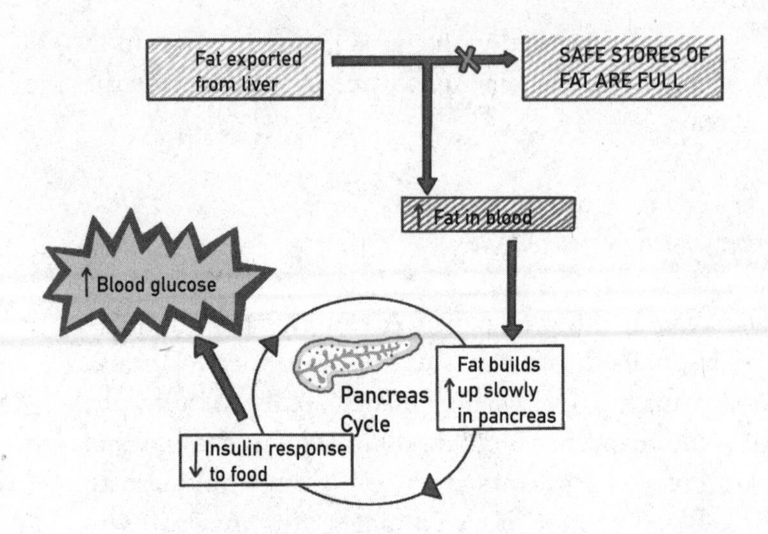

5.2 Second of the twin cycles—the vicious cycle in the pancreas. The normal fat export from the liver can deal with the high liver fat—until the safe storage depot under the skin is full. Then blood levels of fat rise. The pancreas is one of the tissues susceptible to the increased fat. Eventually, after several years, this causes the insulin-producing cells to shut down. Over a short time, blood levels then rise.

Talking about ideas is easy compared with the hard grind of setting down in black and white all the details supported by careful scientific argument. The details could not be imaginary or hopeful. Each had to be linked to sound, published research. Assembling all the detailed scientific justification took six months and then there were further weeks and months while the editor conducted the standard process of asking other scientists to carry out a rigorous scrutiny of the science before deciding whether to accept the article. But eventually the Twin Cycle Hypothesis was published.

The cardinal sin in science is to fall in love with your hypothesis. All scientists know that setting a hypothesis down on paper is the first and very necessary step to discovering how right or wrong it is. The purpose of a hypothesis is to set out in detail what appears to cause what, so that the component ideas can be tested separately. Tested to destruction. Perhaps best not even to say "hypothesis." Try some word substitution. Say "fairytale" instead: it is after all a product of the imagination. I had to say to myself that this was the Twin Cycle Fairytale. That spurred on the process of setting about rigorous testing, with no preconceived ideas. We needed clarity.

A Magic Window Into the Body Using MRI

By one of those great coincidences of scientific life, in 2006 I had just opened a research center based on magnetic resonance (MR). The MRI scan is familiar to all as a routine medical test. It stands for Magnetic Resonance Imaging. But the same technique could be developed by experts to look inside the body and see how different organs were actually functioning. The chemical composition of organs could be measured.

The original idea had been to open the Newcastle MR Center to advance my ongoing research on what happened to food in the body in health and in diabetes, but also to tackle a wide range of questions in all medical specialities: from dementia to muscular dystrophy, from coronary artery disease to arthritis. It had taken me from 2000 to 2004 to raise £5.2 million, and from 2004 to 2006 to design and build the center. However, this was just the groundwork for the critical business. Having the building and the equipment would be useless without expert physicists who could invent the necessary new methods to measure things that had never been measured before. The challenge was to build a world-class MR physics team from scratch.

I had met Andy Blamire, an MR physicist, when we had both worked in the U.S., and was very fortunate in persuading him to move from Oxford to become Professor of MR Physics in Newcastle. We then attracted Dr. Pete Thelwall from the University of Florida and Dr. Kieren Hollingsworth from Cambridge University to join the team. A dream team! And what an exciting era resulted. They devised new techniques for the magnet to answer some of the most important questions of health in every speciality—involving the heart, lung, brain, muscle, kidney, liver, and—of course—the pancreas.

To test the Twin Cycle Hypothesis, we needed to be able to measure the fat content of the liver and pancreas. The liver measurement was quite straightforward to set up, but the pancreas required a brand-new approach. I asked Kieren whether he thought it was possible. He looked up at the ceiling, thought for a few seconds (the longest few seconds in the history of the MR Center), and said "Yes." We were under way. The steeplechase could continue to the next hurdle—finding money to do the work.

Into the Dragons' Den

Medical research is expensive, and a study cannot be carried out without funding. Obtaining the funding is very much like the TV program *Dragons' Den*, in which business ideas are presented to a panel of potential investors. Competition is stiff and the panel members are hard-headed and critical. Scientific grant applications take months of evening and weekend work to prepare and submit. Then the application is sent to half a dozen international experts for their critical review. After that, the Dragons (scientists) on the grant-funding committee discuss both the application itself and the expert opinions. Then they prioritize all applications, and the top few (only around one in 10) are funded. I applied to Diabetes UK, the largest funder of diabetes research in the UK. My application had appeared doomed after scathing expert review and skeptical discussion. What a wild and wacky idea. But just one panel member pointed out that if in the unlikely chance the hypothesis was correct, it could be very important. That person argued that for the modest cost involved it was worth a punt. The application was successful!

The chase began to find out whether the Twin Cycle Hypothesis was wrong—or right. We would do this by asking people with type 2 diabetes to lose a lot of weight. This meant that a sudden drop in food intake would be the only change, with no other complicating factors such as surgery. If their blood glucose stayed high, we would have shown the hypothesis to be wrong and we could go back to the drawing board. If their blood glucose normalized, type 2 diabetes would have been shown to be reversible. Just as important, we would be able to use our MR methods to test whether the mechanisms predicted were correct. We would be able to observe what happened as diabetes changed back to normal—and this would show in reverse how diabetes developed. In other words, we might be able to identify the cause of type 2 diabetes.

Testing the Hypothesis

The Counterpoint Study

Research studies are like people—they need a name and soon take on a life of their own. Most study names are modified acronyms. Our first study had to counteract the effect of fat (triglyceride in scientific jargon) in the pancreas and the liver. What name to choose? Back to the paper and pencil. A page was covered with possibilities. Ideally, the name would be meaningful. One gradually emerged: COUNTERPOINT—COUNTERacting the Pancreatic inhibition Of Insulin secretioN by Triglyceride. Completely irrelevantly, but persuasively for me, the word suggested a favorite novel—Aldous Huxley's *Point Counter Point*. The study was named.

In a working life of testing hypotheses, nothing had paved the way for the starkly clear results of the Counterpoint study. A group of people with very ordinary type 2 diabetes switched to a low-calorie diet, a simple liquid formula diet with non-starchy vegetables that I designed merely as a tool to find out if the twin cycles could be reversed. At the same time, they stopped taking their tablets to decrease blood glucose. Within seven days, their levels of early-morning blood glucose had dropped to normal—just like after bariatric surgery. All the special tests on liver and pancreas confirmed what the hypothesis had predicted—the fat levels inside these organs decreased.

So it seemed our hypothesis might be correct—at least in people with short-duration type 2 diabetes. We had shown that in people who had been diagnosed with type 2 diabetes no more than four years previously, the imagined twin cycles within the liver and pancreas could be reversed to normal. Normal!

The study produced several surprises. The first surprise was seeing just how fatty the liver was in people with type 2 diabetes. At the start of the study, their liver fat level averaged over 13%, which is way above the normal range (up to 5.5%). And to us, at the time, this seemed quite extraordinary in people with ordinary type 2 diabetes, not known to have any liver problems. So this was good going "fatty liver disease." Not a nice condition. It is a sure sign of future heart disease, and it can lead to cirrhosis or worse. Whether you have type 2 diabetes or not, knowing that you almost certainly have too much fat in your liver should be a wake-up call.

The second surprise was how fast the participants' blood glucose fell after they started the very low-calorie diet (see figure 5.3). Equally exciting was the fact that,

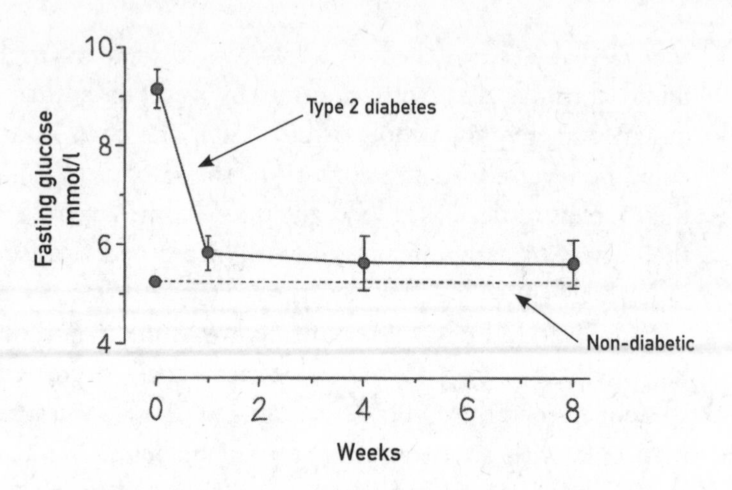

5.3 Within 7 days the glucose level had normalized! The graph above shows the results of the Counterpoint study.

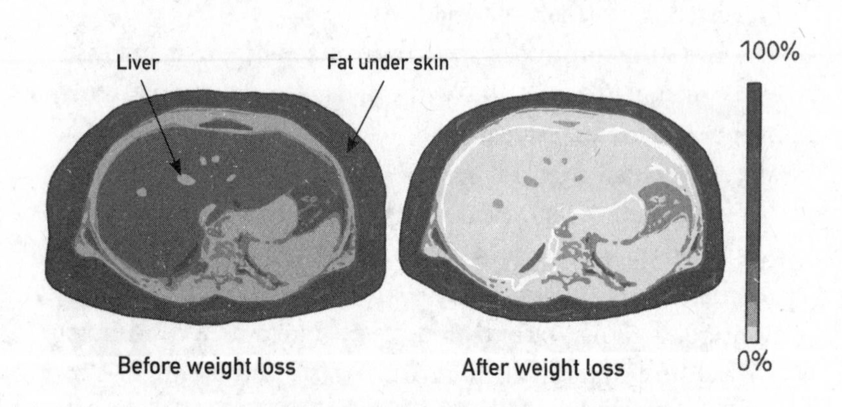

5.4 These pictures are shaded to show the amount of fat in the liver region, with the key for how much % fat on the right. The dark layer of fat under the skin shows up as the most concentrated (100%). But you will see that in the left-hand picture, there is also a very large amount of fat inside the liver itself (36%). After weight loss, the amount of fat in the liver reduces to 2%, as shown by the dramatically lighter shade in the right-hand picture.

within seven days, the insulin resistance of the liver had also vanished, as fat levels fell. We used special tests to measure that directly, and the background insulin levels dropped at the same time. The dramatic change in liver fat during the eight weeks of the study is shown in figure 5.4.

The fat level in the pancreas was high before the diet, but gradually fell to normal. At the same time, the beta cells gradually woke up.

If glucose is injected, the rise in blood glucose normally causes a very sharp increase in insulin production and it is this increase from the background level that is lacking in type 2 diabetes. The normal graph bottom right in figure 5.5 on the next page is from a control group of people without diabetes, but of the same sex and similar age and weight to the group with type 2 diabetes. See how the line rises sharply on this graph, showing the increase in insulin. By contrast, in the graph from the group with type 2 diabetes, see how flat the line is at the start of the study (extreme left), and how, after one week, there is little change, but then by four weeks a sharp increase is evident. And by eight weeks their insulin response is very similar to normal.

Publication of the results of the Counterpoint study in 2011 was followed by considerable interest but also enormous skepticism from experts. After all, there were very good reasons why doctors believed that type 2 diabetes was a lifelong, inevitably progressive condition. Their own experience told them that the condition became more severe over years, needing more and more drugs for

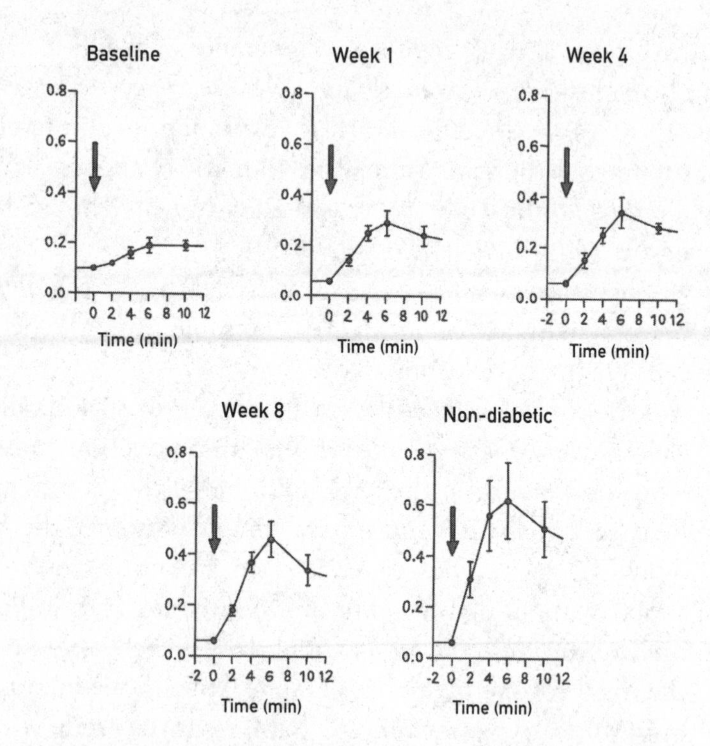

5.5 The insulin-producing cells wake up! The first 4 panels show the response to an increase in blood glucose during the 8 weeks of the Counterpoint study with type 2 diabetes. The 5th graph shows what happens in people without diabetes.

control. Even more persuasively for doctors, large studies on people with type 2 diabetes followed up over many years had clearly shown a steady deterioration in control. After 10 years of living with the disease, as many as one in two people required insulin injections. However, one key thing had been overlooked: that all those observations were made on people who were undergoing progressive weight gain or at best carrying continued excess weight.

That is what happens in practice. After diagnosis, most people become steadily heavier over the years. So it was true that folk with type 2 diabetes tended to get into more and more trouble—but perhaps not inevitably.

Overturning the concept of certain disease progression was too much for most experts. Although a small number immediately accepted the breakthrough, our findings were vehemently opposed, especially by scientists working on the details of studying separate mechanisms that might possibly be causing type 2 diabetes. Scientists have a vast framework of knowledge, but when an idea comes along that removes one of the girders supporting their whole system of beliefs, it is not welcome. In fact, this is not a peculiarity of scientists. It is just the same as in any other walk of life. Try changing a person's beliefs about geography (flat earth?), weather, politics, or anything else merely by providing new facts. Once beliefs are established, facts tend not to get in the way! Bringing about acceptance of change takes persistence and further research.

The Counterpoint Reflections Study

In sharp contrast to the expert disbelief, when the newspapers, radio, and TV reported on the results of Counterpoint, those affected by type 2 diabetes were extremely enthusiastic; they really wanted to find out for themselves whether or not they could escape from the disease. From 2011 onwards, we received a huge number of emails from people asking how they could reverse their own diabetes. To cope, we set up a website containing all the practical information and explaining what they could do to try to improve their condition: https://go.ncl.ac.uk/diabetes-reversal. A second wave of emails then told amazing stories of individuals who had achieved normal blood sugar levels off all their diabetes tablets. Young and old, men and women, rich and poor, living in India, the U.S., South America, Europe, or elsewhere—there was a rich variety of personal stories. This knowledge, collated from people who actually live—or lived—with type 2 diabetes, was analyzed and published as a further scientific paper. Doctors needed to hear from the real experts—those who used to have type 2 diabetes.

And, happily, the data from these real experts confirmed the findings of Counterpoint. The average weight loss achieved by people just armed with the basic information was the same as in Counterpoint—33 pounds. At home and at work, going about their daily lives, people had replicated our research findings. And what emerged was that it was the weight loss that mattered, not the particular diet the participants went on or how they did it. Around half of the group had used a liquid formula diet—as in Counterpoint—and the other half had merely cut back drastically on their normal eating. A high proportion had sought individual advice as advised on our website and had been told by their doctor or diabetes nurse in no uncertain terms not to try to lose weight rapidly. But they were so highly motivated to get rid of their diabetes that they had emailed me on hearing news reports, and understandably they had gone ahead anyway.

Altogether, the reflections told a clear story. First, many people with type 2 diabetes really hated their condition and would go to any lengths to escape from it. Most doctors and nurses did not know that. Second, motivated people could return to normal glucose control when simply provided with clear information on how to do it.

All of a sudden, the research broadened out from its initial goal. I had set out to find out what caused type 2 diabetes. I had hoped to clarify the mechanisms involved and perhaps point a way forward for future treatment. Job done. But the tool developed to test the hypothesis—a low-calorie liquid diet—seemed to be a real-world solution for many people who could use it to get rid of their own diabetes.

Encouraged by this "proof of the pudding" (or maybe proof of no pudding), we pressed on with more research.

Counterbalance

Is it possible to enjoy long-term remission from type 2 diabetes while eating normally? This was the most important question that faced us. After rapid weight loss, could the body remain in balance and control blood glucose levels normally on a return to eating ordinary food? The original Counterpoint study had shown that we could indeed <u>COUNTER</u> <u>P</u>ancreatic inhibition <u>O</u>f <u>I</u>nsulin secretio<u>N</u> by <u>T</u>riglyceride. The acronym had proved true, at least in the short term. We called the second major study

Counterbalance. That stood for COUNTERacting BetA cell failure by Long-term Action to Normalize Calorie intakE. A bit long, but it did what it said on the tin!

Under the guidance of Dr. Sarah Steven, just like its older sister, this study took on a life of its own. In Counterbalance, rapid weight loss was first achieved in eight weeks using exactly the same diet as Counterpoint; and then we introduced normal foods in a stepwise fashion over two weeks. We had learned from the Counterpoint pioneers that when they stopped the one-package-per-meal diet it was tough to readjust to deciding what food to eat.

Sarah gave individualized advice on how much to eat and what foods to avoid and saw each person once per month. Over the following six months, our research participants kept their average weight rock steady. At the end of this, everyone who had got rid of their diabetes after the initial weight loss remained non-diabetic. Just like in Counterpoint, the pancreas woke up after weight loss and started to produce insulin normally again, this time for nine months after the start of the study. Important for understanding how this happened, liver fat remained really low, at 2%, and their pancreas fat fell to even safer levels. Diabetes had gone away and stayed away.

Falko Sniehotta, professor of psychology at Newcastle, and his team carried out tests to identify the main barriers to success, and also what advice was most helpful for people to succeed in losing weight and keeping it off. The results of this have informed the information provided in Chapters 7 and 8.

Did the duration of diabetes make a difference?

Yes. The longer the duration of type 2 diabetes, the lower the likelihood was of getting back to normal glucose control. But never say never. Counterbalance determined the betting odds of achieving remission of diabetes. This decreased from close to a dead certainty soon after diagnosis to 50/50 in the first 10 years, then much lower chances after that. Betting odds are a guide to how likely it is you will win. But they just indicate average chance. From time to time, the 100-to-1 outsider romps home, and the results certainly did not mean that nobody with very long-duration type 2 diabetes could benefit. Some people living with type 2 diabetes for more than 20 years have successfully reversed to normal. Two individuals in Newcastle who had 24 years of diabetes and poor blood glucose control, on two kinds of tablets every day, have returned to normal off tablets after losing over 33 pounds in weight. The important message is that it is never too late to attempt to reverse your diabetes, although success is not guaranteed.

The Counterbalance results were all the more remarkable because the group who reversed their diabetes during the study had not become slim. The average BMI (Body Mass Index) had started at 33, and it decreased to 29. So approximately half of the group were still technically obese. But they continued to be free of diabetes. They were carrying more fat than they really needed, but for them, it stayed in the safety of the fat layer under the skin and did not redistribute to clog up the liver and pancreas. At least over the total study duration of around nine months.

Wow! A new world of understanding of type 2 diabetes was opening up. Counterbalance confirmed that the process of reversing diabetes could potentially be used as a normal treatment for people with type 2.

The Pancreas Study

One of the most controversial aspects of the Twin Cycle Hypothesis was that the pancreatic beta cells were predicted to be struggling as a result of too much fat inside and around them. When the Counterpoint results were announced, this discussion became important. Some experts pointed out—quite reasonably—that the recovery of the cells may have been only indirectly related to weight loss. Maybe the waking up was coincidental and due to something else. Was the fall in pancreas fat merely because of the weight loss itself? Perhaps fat levels decreased in all organs after weight loss. Well, if so, it would happen in people who did not have type 2 diabetes too. This was something we could test: was the fall in pancreas fat something special that happened in people with diabetes, or would it happen to people without diabetes too?

The easiest way to do this was to compare what happened after bariatric surgery. Weight loss after the operation would be the same whether or not individuals had type 2 diabetes. We could compare what happened to pancreas fat in each group.

Bariatric surgery is highly effective at causing weight

loss. Unsurprisingly, if your stomach was suddenly reduced to the size of your thumb, you would lose weight too. In the North East of England, we have one of the largest bariatric surgery services, with superb surgeons. Mr. Peter Small and Mr. Sean Woodcock were hugely helpful in planning a collaborative research study. With funding from the European Foundation for the Study of Diabetes, the Pancreas study got under way.

Participants with and without diabetes were of similar weight and age, and there was a male/female balance. Peter and Sean did their magic: everyone had a stomach bypass operation, performed entirely via telescopes and tubes (laparoscopic surgery), and, after eight weeks, both those with and without diabetes had lost around 29 pounds.

This study confirmed that the level of fat inside the pancreas was abnormally high in people with type 2 diabetes, but that this high level dropped when food intake was suddenly decreased. In contrast, it did not fall at all in people without diabetes during the eight weeks of this study. We can now be reasonably sure that the fall in fat levels inside the pancreas is related to the diabetes itself and linked to recovery of normal insulin secretion. Absolute certainty in medicine is rare.

The Pancreas study also allowed us to test another idea. As mentioned earlier, some people thought that bariatric surgery had a "special" effect in improving blood glucose control via incretin hormones. This appeared unlikely to me on theoretical grounds, but now we had a chance to find out if I was right or wrong. The people with diabetes awaiting bariatric surgery were randomly divided into two groups. Half had the bariatric surgery, with tests before and one week later. The other half had a week of a very low-calorie diet with tests before and after (and only then had their surgery). Was it all about the sudden decrease in food intake? Was there any special effect of bariatric surgery via the incretin hormones?

Sarah Steven devised a special, small test meal that could be managed by people after bariatric surgery. In the surgery group, because of the stomach bypass, the small test meal very rapidly went into the small intestine. After the surgery, there was a huge (seven-fold) increase in incretin hormones. But the insulin response was identical after the meal whether people had undergone surgery or just an equivalent drop in calorie intake. The effect of bariatric surgery on the incretin hormones was real but had nothing at all to do with the sudden return to normal of blood glucose levels. This was merely an effect of the drastic decrease in food intake. A similar study carried out in America found identical results. Whether food intake is voluntarily decreased by diet or enforced by surgery, the results on glucose levels are the same. Once again, careful testing had yielded a clear result.

DiRECT—The Diabetes Remission Clinical Trial

Our early studies had set the stage and explained what was going on in the body, but it became clear during Counterbalance that what had been developed as a tool to test the hypothesis (the low-calorie diet) might be useful in routine care. It was actually liked by people with type 2 diabetes, even though they found it challenging. The question was, would it work in real life? So far, the treatment had only been carried out in research centers by specialist doctors on patients who were motivated to join the study. Type 2 diabetes is usually managed in primary care. We had to find out whether the staff who provided the routine care for people with diabetes could help everyone achieve and maintain substantial weight loss.

There were other big questions waiting to be answered. After going into remission, would diabetes stay away for at least two years? Although we knew of many people who had been free of the disease for longer than this after weight loss, only a formal study on a large group of people could give an answer that would convince other doctors. And would the lower levels of fat in the liver and pancreas be maintained with normal function of these organs?

My application to fund such a study was rejected by Diabetes UK. But it was turned down constructively. At the same meeting, a separate application had been discussed. That was from Professor Mike Lean, an internationally renowned expert on obesity and nutrition. At that time, he was testing a low-calorie liquid diet, followed by a structured weight maintenance program, in obesity. This trial was being conducted in routine primary care. Some months before, he had asked me to help with his application to expand the trial to tackle type 2 diabetes, so our names were already linked. Both our applications were rejected—but with an inspired bit of thinking.

The Grants Committee asked Mike and me to collaborate on a combined, much larger single study. Mike's specialist knowledge about obesity and links with primary care could be combined with my experience of reversing type 2 diabetes. Work at the interface of scientific areas can be transformational, and we did not hesitate in taking on the challenge.

We planned DiRECT with the aim of achieving a clinically important result. We decided that releasing one in five people from diabetes, off all tablets, at one year would be very useful—important for each individual, and important for the costs of providing health care. The size of the study was planned on this assumption. Mike had used an almost identical overall approach (known as Counterweight Plus) to mine in primary care but with four shakes per day and no vegetables for the weight loss phase, and we decided to use this to minimize variation in the trial.

In fact, we found that one person in two of the weight loss group had no diabetes at one year, and no longer needed tablets or injections. After two years, the proportion in remission was still over one third—far better than we had planned, even for the one-year mark. Of those who were in remission from their diabetes at one year, the vast majority remained diabetes-free at two years. Even more remarkably, if people maintained weight loss of more than 22 pounds for two years, then two out of three remained in remission.

The joy of those people at having got rid of their disease was in itself a pleasure to behold for the whole DiRECT team. Also, the health service cost savings were potentially eye-watering. The major costs of diabetes are actually in treating the complications of the disease, and DiRECT observed fewer of these in the weight loss group compared with those treated according to the conventional official guidelines. Longer-term follow-up will be important to obtain hard information on the exact level of reduction of complications, but the writing is clearly on the wall.

As part of the study, detailed metabolic studies were done on those people who lived in or around Tyneside. The studies showed that everyone who lost weight achieved normalization of liver fat and rates of export of liver fat to the rest of the body. Pancreas fat levels fell. These benefits were seen in everyone who lost weight—even in those who remained diabetic. We had not anticipated that. For the first time, we saw that the ultimate deciding factor in achieving remission of type 2 diabetes was inside the beta cell itself. Getting rid of the fat was necessary, but not sufficient. It looked as though the beta cells in the people who did not get rid of their diabetes may have been too badly affected by the excess fat. We had already discovered that longer-duration type 2 diabetes was much less likely to reverse completely, and this explained why some people do not achieve remission.

There was a small number of people who had been in remission at one year but regained most of the weight lost by two years. They unfortunately slipped back into diabetes, despite the best efforts of the team. But this provided a great scientific opportunity. We were able to watch the diabetes as it developed. That had never been done before. And the predictions of the Twin Cycle Hypothesis were confirmed—as liver fat export increased, pancreas fat increased and then insulin production failed in the beta cells.

From Hypothesis to Action

It had taken from 2006, when the Twin Cycle Hypothesis was conceived, through 2011, when the mechanisms by which diabetes returned to normal were proven, to December 2017. That is when the first-year results of DiRECT were announced. The concept that too much fat inside vital organs caused type 2 diabetes was gradually gaining ground. But the demonstration of the successful application of this knowledge by routine health care staff precipitated game, set, and match. In June 2018, the American Diabetes Association changed its policy and officially recognized that remission of type 2 diabetes was a desirable aim of treatment. That same year, both NHS England and NHS Scotland announced funding for the weight-loss-based approach to achieving remission of type 2 diabetes. Slow, gradual change in the belief system had brought about change in policy.

After the first report of the Counterpoint study (2011), many people had asked why remission of type 2 diabetes was not already funded by the NHS. It is natural to wonder why not, if you have seen your own diabetes disappear. Should roll-out into routine clinical practice have happened more quickly? Probably not. It is critically important that major changes in medical concepts are challenged and thoroughly tested before acceptance. Scientists and doctors have to be skeptical to ensure that medicine—health care—moves forward on a carefully tested, solid basis.

This is the beginning of a story, not the end. Much is yet to be discovered, especially about the best way to keep weight off in the long term. The detailed research had shown that type 2 diabetes was not a complex, heterogeneous condition but a simple condition happening in a heterogeneous group of people. At least we have moved from hypothesis, through scientific proof, to further studies and on to practical advice for all comers. There is now a new understanding of type 2 diabetes.

Why Does Fat Switch Off Your Beta Cells?

And so to the final unanswered question in our detective story about the missing beta cells. From Counterpoint, Counterbalance, and DiRECT, we had learned that removing the fat from the pancreas would usually allow the beta cells to wake up and start producing insulin normally. We had come a long way, but our work in real people could not show precisely what might be happening inside the beta cells to allow this miracle to happen. For clarity on this puzzle, which had remained unsolved for decades, we have to thank Professor Domenico Accili in New York and other scientists including Dr. Anne Clark in Oxford and Professor James Shaw in Newcastle, whose research has shown the mechanism by which fat affects beta cells to cause diabetes.

Beta cells are exquisitely sensitive to the supply of energy as their special business is making insulin when fuel is coming in. Excess fat causes stress in the beta cells of some people—those who are susceptible to type 2 diabetes. Because of sustained fat attack, their beta cells take cover by hunkering down and going into survival mode. This is intensified once diabetes develops and glucose levels rise; and to survive, the beta cells switch off the genes needed for insulin production. They will just sit there, concentrating on their own survival with no spare capacity to serve the best interests of the rest of the body.

Because the insulin production had been switched off in many beta cells, the cells were not missing but merely not functioning. This process of a cell losing its specialist function is called "de-differentiation," because specialist cells acquire their special function by differentiating from basic cells. The process is illustrated in figure 5.6.

Back in 2008, the Twin Cycle Hypothesis predicted that the beta cell problem in type 2 diabetes should be a reversible process. We now know why removing the excess fat allows resumption of business as usual—the switch-off of those genes for insulin production is reversible if the level of fat inside the cell is decreased. But if it continues too long, the apparatus to make insulin seems to become ineffective.

But hang on, you may say: How does all this square with the observation described at the start of this chapter that around half of the beta cells seemed to have died? This is simple. Scientists recognize beta cells under the microscope by staining them with a marker that shows the insulin content. Because the insulin production had been switched off in many beta cells these were not detectable under the microscope. The cells were still alive, but you may say had "gone undercover." The cells were not missing but merely hidden from view.

No murder, but just a dormant state. If asked, perhaps a beta cell in type 2 diabetes would quote Mark Twain: "Rumors of my death have been much exaggerated!"

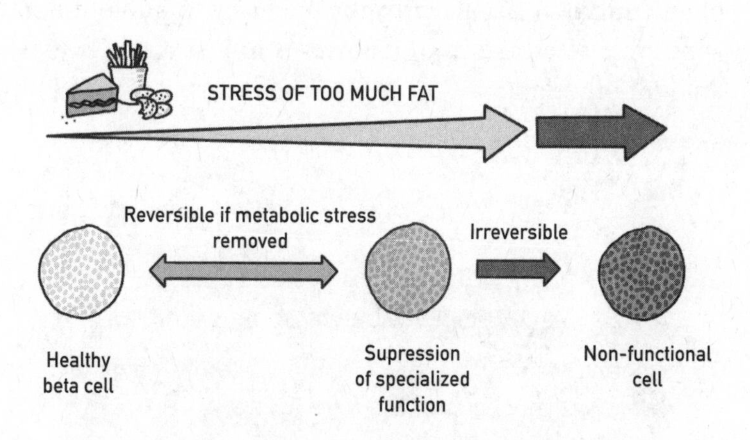

5.6 Too much fat inside insulin-producing cells—in susceptible people—gradually causes them to stop making insulin normally. This is a reversible process in the early years of type 2 diabetes, but if it continues too long then it becomes irreversible.

The fascinating story does not end there. Individuals with type 2 diabetes vary in their ability to withstand the metabolic onslaught of excess fat. Some people can still return to non-diabetic levels of blood glucose control after more than 20 years of type 2 diabetes. Some seem to lose this capacity relatively rapidly. In other words, different people have differing levels of beta cell durability in the face of fat attack. Those people who were able to reverse their type 2 diabetes after 24 years must have had susceptible, but exceptionally durable beta cells. It looks very much as though there is a different set of genes that determines the durability of the beta cell. In years to come, we will no doubt see further developments on this front.

But the bottom line for a person with type 2 diabetes of any duration is: currently, the only way to find out if it is possible to escape from diabetes is to lose a substantial amount of weight.

Quick Read

- The Twin Cycle Hypothesis tied together the best available evidence about control of blood glucose
- The predictions of the hypothesis were tested in a series of studies
- Type 2 diabetes was shown to be initiated by too much glucose and fat being produced by the liver

- The excess fat causes pancreatic beta cells to lose their special ability to make insulin
- Defects in both the liver and pancreas can be corrected by substantial weight loss
- The alleged murder never happened: when beta cells are prevented from making insulin they cannot be detected under the microscope but are still living

6

The Personal Fat Threshold

News items about type 2 diabetes are frequently accompanied by pictures of very large people, creating an impression that type 2 diabetes is caused by obesity. Even doctors sometimes state that the type 2 diabetes epidemic is due to obesity. This leads to the common assumption that if an individual has type 2 diabetes, they must be obese and it is all their own fault.

But the truth is that the vast majority of very heavy people do not have type 2 diabetes, and only half of all people developing the condition have a BMI in the obese range.

Let's have a reality check.

Why Have I Got Type 2 Diabetes?

René Laennec was the famous French doctor who invented the stethoscope. He used to say to his students: "Listen to your patients. They are giving you the diagnosis." He was not talking about listening to the heart or lungs with his new invention. He was talking about the most important skill of a doctor—informed listening. Listening to the story a patient tells about why they have sought medical advice can lead to an understanding of the sort of disease that has caused their symptoms. This is the basis of clinical diagnosis. It is a message still relevant today.

When the results of our first study on reversing type 2 diabetes were reported by the newspapers and on television in 2011, we were inundated by emails from people with diabetes telling us about their condition, how long they had had it, what complications they had experienced, and whether it was well controlled. Many people just wanted to learn how they could get rid of their diabetes. But there was a substantial minority who emailed to say that they were not overweight but had still developed type 2 diabetes. Many doctors will be familiar with this phenomenon, and be accustomed to their patients asking why this is the case: "Why have I got type 2 diabetes when my friends are all fatter than me and they don't have it?"

At first, this might seem to be at odds with the Twin Cycle Hypothesis described in Chapter 5. That starts off with the idea that eating more than the body requires over a long period of time is necessary for the condition to develop.

For me, an early insight into what may be going on in type 2 diabetes had come some years earlier from a non-obese person who had the disease. Let's call this person Mark. Mark was outraged that diabetes had happened to him, a person who was not obese—not even overweight—and had come to me to see if there was any way of getting rid of it. We performed some blood tests, which showed that his liver was not as healthy as it should have been, and this caught my attention. All of this was before the Twin Cycle Hypothesis was developed, but I already knew that in type 2 diabetes, these particular tests were often around the upper border of normal—or a little bit high. I also knew, from our research, that there were high levels of fat in the liver in type 2 diabetes and that this caused the liver to make too much glucose.

I therefore reasoned that the high levels of liver fat might be causing a problem, which was in turn leading to type 2 diabetes. If this was true, then we possibly had a plan of action. Why not suggest substantial weight loss as a possible way of getting rid of Mark's liver fat and thereby potentially improving the control of his diabetes too? This unconventional advice was offered with no guarantees of success; it was just a possible way to return to health and, at best, fulfilled the vital criterion laid down so long ago by Hippocrates: "At least do no harm." But Mark was adamant that he wanted to get back to normal or as near normal as he could and said he would try it.

So "normal-weight" Mark lost weight. His BMI went down from 24 to just below 20. And the diabetes went away.

Interestingly, it was not just the blood glucose first thing in the morning that normalized. It was also the level of blood glucose two hours after swallowing a test glucose drink. Clearly, something else was going on as well as the predicted liver changes. And that something was likely to be a change in the function of the pancreas. Which came as a bit of a surprise.

Had Mark become abnormally thin? Not at all—for him. In fact, he had merely decreased his weight to what it was in his early 20s. It seemed that he had accumulated more fat than he could store safely, and he had certainly been unable to cope with the amount of fat in his liver. That had brought about a situation that his body had not been able to manage. His weight had been too high *for him*—even though it was unremarkable compared with what was "normal" for most people. The whole episode set me thinking about what was normal for one person, and how this was not represented by the normal range for the whole population.

So, fast-forward to 2011, when the dramatic results of Counterpoint were published. As mentioned before, among the emails we received were a fair number from people with type 2 diabetes with a normal BMI. Because of the good effect on Mark and the Counterpoint results, it seemed reasonable to provide the information that losing weight in such circumstances could get rid of type 2 diabetes. In responding to medical questions by email, a doctor can only put forward information and not personal medical advice. It is essential not to get in the way of the person's own doctor. So we limited ourselves to providing this information and advising people to discuss it with their own doctor or nurse.

You may guess what happened next. We started to receive emails reporting return to normal glucose levels from this group of "normal-weight" people. Many had followed the recommendation to discuss the weight loss plan in advance with their doctor or nurse—and had been rebuffed. Don't do it, they were told in no uncertain terms, it is unhealthy to lose weight as your BMI is already in the normal range. But in most of these people the desire to escape from type 2 diabetes was so strong that they ignored this well-meaning advice. One of them was a journalist, and he wrote about his experience in the *Guardian* (see Bibliography). His article helped a considerable number of people.

In many walks of life as well as in medicine, limits are set for what is normal. But time and again during my scientific career, I have found that such limits can be too restrictive. There really is no one size that fits all. Perhaps as a society we need to shake off the shackles of political correctness. A normal BMI is defined as less than 25. But just look at your fellow human beings in the street. We come in all shapes and sizes. What if those who do not look chubby on the outside actually have too much fat on the inside? To me, years ago when I first met Mark, this notion was not new. It had previously been described by several names, including "TOFI"—Thin Outside, Fat Inside. But now, thanks to Mark and various respondents who wrote in, I knew we were on to something: maybe people who were not overweight but had developed type 2 diabetes had been thinner when they were in their 20s, and their weight gain was "invisible."

Back to the drawing board. How could these concepts be captured in a few words? Everyone is an individual. Fact. Could it be that each person might have an individual level of tolerance for fat build-up in the body? The Personal Fat Threshold concept was born.

Looking at the Population

In the 1970s and 1980s, the population of the UK was considerably lighter than at present. In fact, reliable information from surveys carried out in 1980 and 2012 reveals that the average weight of both men and women increased during those three decades by 22 pounds—yes, 22 pounds! In 1980, the general population had an average BMI of 24. Can you remember what folk looked like then? Look at this photo of a Newcastle street scene taken then, to refresh that memory. Let's consider what has happened in only 32 years.

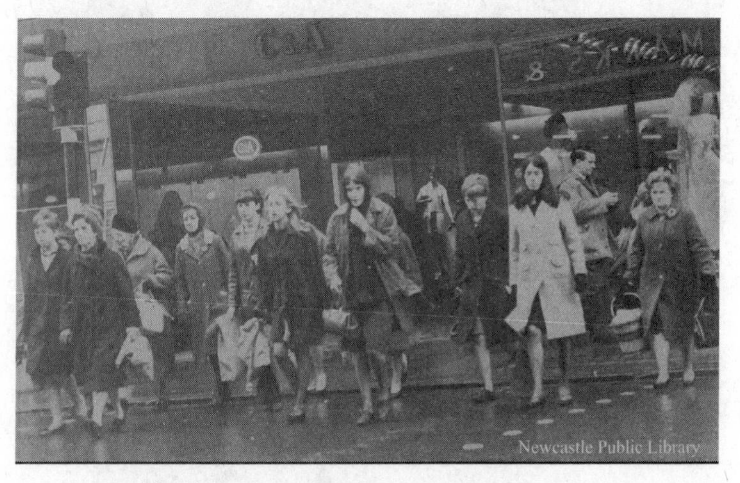

6.1 People on the street in Newcastle in the late 1970s. It was rare to see an overweight person.

Figure 6.2 on the next page shows the BMI levels of the adult population of England and Wales as they were in 1980. Everyone with a BMI over 30 would be labeled "obese."

At the time, this amounted to about one in every 14 people, or 7%.

In 2012, this survey was repeated—see figure 6.3. The proportion of the population with a BMI over 30 had shot up to one in four people, or 25%. 25%!

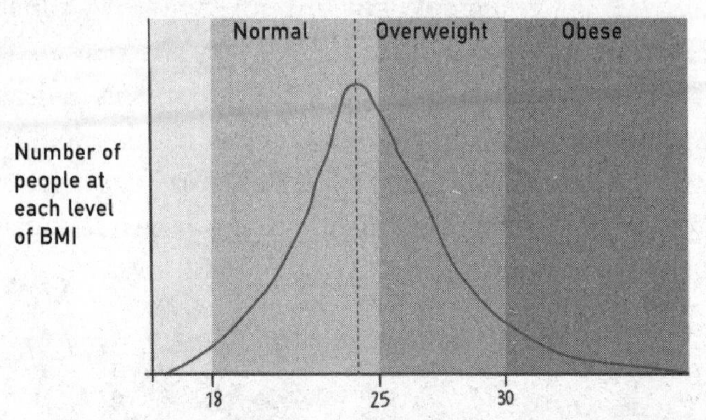

6.2 How many people were at each level of BMI in 1980? The most common BMI was 24 (dotted line). Very few people had a BMI of over 30 and would be classified as obese.

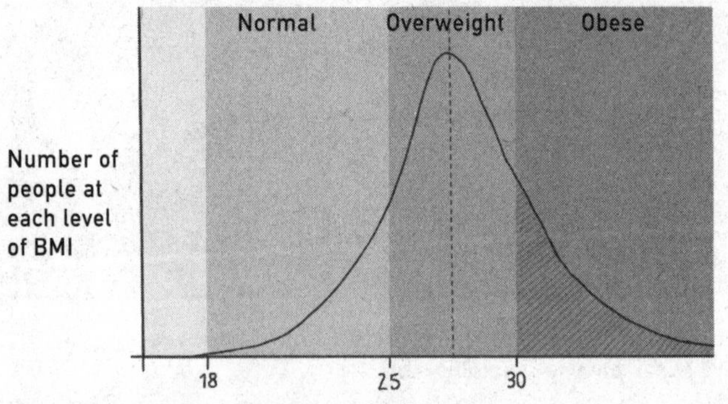

6.3 By 2012, obesity had become much commoner (shaded area). But that is not the biggest change. The mountain had moved—almost everyone had increased in weight. The shape of the curve is similar to the 1980 graph and the most common BMI had become 27 (dotted line).

The headline news sounds shocking: that between 1980 and 2012, the rate of obesity in the adult population of England and Wales had increased from one in 14 to one in four. What was wrong with these people? "They" needed to be sorted out, so the argument went. It has to be said again that most discussions about the rising incidence of obesity miss the point. Attention is riveted on those who have a BMI over 30. Certainly, this is obesity by the widely accepted, fixed definition. But look again at the graphs. The change in weight is not restricted to those who became obese. It is not them and us. We have all become heavier.

- People who used to have a BMI of 35 now have a BMI of 38. They are more obese.
- People who used to have a BMI of 29 now have a BMI of 31 and have become obese.
- People who used to have a BMI of 24 now have a BMI of 27 and have become overweight.
- Thin people have increased their BMI from 19 to 22 and are still defined as normal.

This summary is useful to understand the wider picture, but reflects only the average weight gain. Of course, some people gained more than others. Appetite is largely genetically determined, and yours reflects your luck of the draw when your genes were inherited. Those born with the most active appetites, people superbly tuned for survival during food scarcity, tend to put on the most weight in any given environment. There are other influences on appetite, but here we are talking about effects seen in populations. The environment (largely food availability) determines the average weight of any population. But whether an individual is heavier or lighter than others with the same access to food depends largely on their genes.

The reality is that the environment in which we live has changed, and the population is changing as a consequence. This was neatly captured in a few words in a *Lancet* article in 2002: "The obesity epidemic is due to normal people, doing normal things, in an abnormal environment." Some enthusiasts for personal action on health would dispute this view, arguing that we are not the slaves of our environment, that health is a personal responsibility, and letting our weight get too high is irresponsible. However, this view does not recognize that aspiring to best health is not the number one concern day to day for many people. For those in particularly fortunate circumstances, much time and thought can be devoted every day to keeping weight down or taking exercise. But for the majority, life intervenes—illness in the family, a leaking roof, financial problems, work demands—and what we eat, when, how and how much, is not a primary focus of attention. Nor does it have to be to survive: in our time-poor modern world, the constant availability of food, being surrounded by others eating at any time, the acceptability of eating while in the street, all enable us to fuel up mindlessly. Like it or not, most of our lives run on autopilot.

All creatures are affected by their environment, and humans are no different. And when the environment provides something immediately pleasurable, successfully fighting against it is a minority pastime. It really should be a no-brainer.

The Personal Fat Threshold—Let's Hear It for the Individual

The graphs on the next page illustrate that the average BMI has increased—the whole mountain has moved (compare figures 6.2 and 6.3). But while it is shocking that the population has become so much heavier, this is population science, not medicine. We are all individuals. Doctors have just one patient in front of them in a consultation. So let's imagine some of these individuals.

Panel A shows individuals according to their BMI. The overall information is similar to the population distribution graph, figure 6.2, on page 136, but instead of just a smooth line telling us about the whole population, individuals are shown. Each dark gray dot is one person with type 2 diabetes. For this group, you will see that the commonest BMI is around 27. The graph enables us to see what might happen to each person with diabetes over time. For instance, what if they all lost 33 pounds in weight?

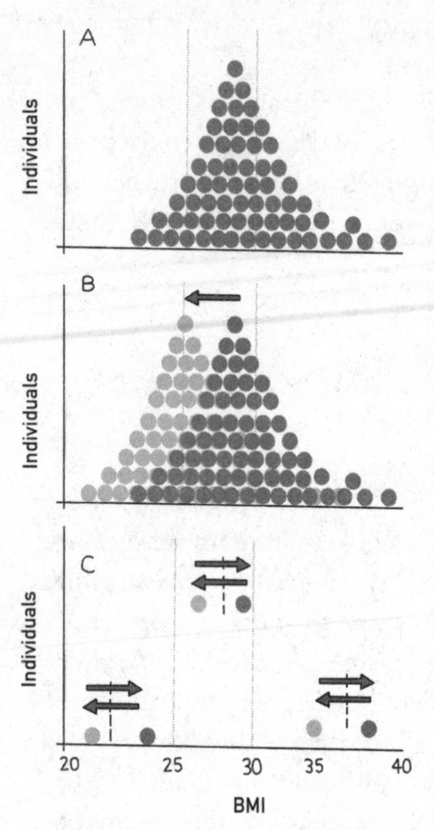

6.4
Each dot is one person, showing their BMI. Normal BMI is between the dotted lines. The most common BMI is 28 in this group of people with type 2 diabetes.

If each person lost 33 pounds, they are likely to become non-diabetic. The same individuals are now shown in light gray as well. There has been a big population shift in BMI, with the most common now being 25.

Let's look at just 3 individuals. One is free of diabetes with a BMI of 34—but this is far higher than the person who started off with diabetes at a BMI of 24. What happened is that each person has crossed their own Personal Fat Threshold.

The middle panel shows the same individuals, but after each had lost 33 pounds in weight. Assume that everyone reversed their diabetes. Each dot has changed from dark gray to light gray to indicate this. What has happened is that the mountain has moved to the left. Every single individual has changed their BMI. If we were just looking at the usual smooth curve for a population, the pundits would say: "Just look at the fall in obesity rate—from

36% to less than 7%." This approach focuses on the fixed cut-off for obesity—a BMI of over 30. And once again, the important point would have been overlooked.

In the lower panel, we can see what happened to just three of these individuals. Let's call them Jack, Mary, and Harry (right to left). Jack lost 33 pounds, his BMI changed from 38 to 35, and he became non-diabetic. Mary lost 33 pounds, shifted her BMI from 29 to 26, and also became non-diabetic. Harry started with BMI 24 and lost weight to BMI 21 and he became non-diabetic too.

Just for a moment, we could go back to the population experts and ask them what has happened. They would say: "Nothing had happened. Just look at the data. Jack is still obese (BMI over 30). Mary is still overweight (BMI 25–30). Harry is still normal weight." You can see how fixed cut-offs that put people into watertight categories can be misleading. The message is: if you are seeking advice about your own health, do not consult a population expert! That said, they do a great job in describing populations, and when a whole population becomes heavier, as is happening in many countries today, the number of people developing type 2 diabetes increases.

Now let's imagine that each of our individuals, Jack, Mary, and Harry, regain all the weight they had lost and their BMIs increase by three to return to 38, 29, and 24 respectively. Their BMIs are still very different, but each of them will have crossed their personal limit of tolerance for carrying excess fat. The capacity to store fat safely in the tissue under the skin varies considerably between individuals.

Some people have positively athletic fat tissue under the skin, which can handle anything thrown at it, with apparently endless storage capacity. Lucky people, we might say from a metabolic point of view. Of course, if they acquire more and more fat it may look excessive, but it is all locked up safely. As we have seen, the metabolic trouble starts when fat can no longer be stored safely and has to be stowed away somewhere else.

Insight from a Classic Research Study

One research study stands out as having influenced knowledge on type 2 diabetes more than any other. Twenty-five years ago, it also profoundly changed how doctors treated the condition. It asked the main question: does better control of blood glucose prevent long-term complications of diabetes? The United Kingdom Prospective Diabetes Study, usually abbreviated to UKPDS, enrolled people with newly diagnosed type 2 diabetes between 1977 and 1991. The main findings emerged in 1998.

It was the brainchild of Dr. Robert Turner at Oxford University. He battled against seemingly impossible odds to keep the study going by obtaining funding throughout the 20 years of the main study. He was an independent thinker, an excellent doctor, and had formidable determination. But over and above all of that, he could attract and maintain a loyal group of doctors scattered across the UK. He was a remarkable man, and needed all his attributes to launch, execute, and complete the study. In 1975,

Dr. Turner and his team were joined by another enlightened medical academic, Dr.—now Professor—Rury Holman. He was also instrumental in making the trial work from conception to completion (1977–97). In 2012, he agreed to collaborate with me in reanalyzing some of the old UKPDS data to test the Personal Fat Threshold idea: was it possible that individuals had a certain level of fat stores that was safe for them but different from others'?

UKPDS was by far the largest "randomized" trial in diabetes at the time. Randomized means that people were assigned at random: either to the intensive treatment group or to a "control" group. This design is important as it minimizes the risk of getting a misleading result. If people choose which treatment group they are to join it is highly likely it would influence the findings, and any differences measured at the end could merely reflect this. Any bias between the groups would mean that the results may not be due to the treatment given to that group but to something else unidentified—such as motivation, personal experience of previous medical issues or background beliefs about illness. The participants in the control group in UKPDS were treated as usual (diet, eventually tablets and rarely insulin) but those in the intensive group were treated with tablets or insulin as needed with the revolutionary aim of keeping fasting blood glucose below 6mmol/l.

At the time UKPDS was designed, such randomized trials were rare in studying any disease. But Robert Turner was a pioneer who wanted to establish new knowledge that was beyond criticism. There has been no other study quite like UKPDS. A total of 5,102 people with diabetes took part in it. Twenty years later, it produced absolutely dramatic information. It found that better control of blood glucose brought about very worthwhile reductions in all the complications of diabetes—eye, nerve, kidney, foot, heart, and brain. That was big news. At the time, many doctors thought that diabetic complications happened irrespective of how well the blood glucose level was controlled. This old belief took a very long time to be replaced, but today there is universal acceptance of the link between blood glucose control and the risk of long-term complications.

The research also showed that blood glucose levels rose steadily over the years, irrespective of whether people were in the control or intensive group. Type 2 diabetes seemed to get inexorably worse. Everyone appeared to need increasing numbers of tablets and by 10 years, half had been started on insulin injections. This clear proof of steady deterioration was eventually accepted worldwide, reinforcing the simple observation of most specialists in diabetes: people had type 2 diabetes for life and blood glucose levels steadily got worse. Subsequently, all this coalesced into a rather gloomy message: it became a fixed belief that type 2 diabetes inevitably progressed and sooner or later insulin treatment would be needed; everyone went downhill however energetically tablets were prescribed. You may have been introduced to the gloom and doom when you were diagnosed. Nonetheless, UKPDS brought about a worldwide revolution in knowledge about how type 2 diabetes appeared to be best treated.

The importance of UKPDS to this chapter, though,

involves a different matter. In UKPDS, what was the *weight* of this group of people with newly diagnosed diabetes? The average BMI was 27. That is not high at all. It is in the lower part of the overweight range, far short of obesity. Approximately one third of these people developing very ordinary type 2 diabetes had a completely normal BMI—less than 25.

In fact, the distribution of the dark gray dots in figure 6.4 exactly reflects the BMI of the people who enrolled in UKPDS.

It may seem strange, given the way type 2 diabetes is portrayed and reported on now, but back in the 1970s and early 1980s it was accepted that obesity had nothing directly to do with the cause of type 2 diabetes. Several well-known studies seemed to show this. As a young doctor, I myself reviewed all the best evidence and published a summary concluding that there was no link! How could this be? We now can see that the few obese people around at the time would have had an increased risk of type 2 diabetes but the effect overall was undetectable because of the small total number of obese people.

Where was the obesity in UKPDS? Good question. The nature of type 2 diabetes was just the same, then as now. But individuals in the background population were very different—they were quite simply less heavy.

It is somewhat paradoxical, then, that the group of relatively slim people who took part in UKPDS has provided the majority of today's conventional knowledge of type 2 diabetes. Such are the pitfalls of accepted beliefs: because type 2 has come to be associated with being overweight, even most diabetes experts today will look at the study's results and believe their assumptions confirmed. What they may not appreciate is that the population studied in UKPDS looked very different from any average group of people with type 2 diabetes today. Only one in 14 people back then was obese and, astonishingly, from today's perspective, one in three had a normal BMI.

Today, even specialists refer to type 2 diabetes as a disease of obesity. And yet, at the time of diagnosis, still only 50% of type 2 diabetics are obese (i.e., have a BMI over 30). The other 50% are non-obese. Also, one in 10 people are in the normal range of BMI (under 25) at the time of diagnosis. These figures are for people of white European ethnicity. In people of South Asian or Far Eastern ethnicity, the number with type 2 diabetes yet a normal BMI is much higher.

A Population Shift

Remember the figures mentioned before—on average back in 1980 both men and women weighed 33 pounds less than they do today and had an average BMI of 24. Turn back to page 135 and try to find obese people in the photograph of a Newcastle street scene from that era. Today the background population has a BMI of 27, and finding obese people in a current photograph would not be difficult because the whole population has increased in weight.

Why Were the Majority of UKPDS Participants Non-Obese?

As we have seen, for any given level of BMI, some people may have quite a lot of fat stored under the skin and not much inside the stomach cavity, whereas others may have ordinary amounts under the skin but a lot inside. The big advantage of using magnetic resonance methods to study how we handle food is that the inside structures of the body are routinely visible and accessible for measuring content of fat, glycogen, and other goodies. Look at figures 2.6 and 2.7 to see just how different people look inside.

The fat stored inside the stomach cavity is not necessarily bad in itself. But it is an indicator that the normal safe storage depot under the skin is full, so fat is building up anywhere it can, including inside the body's organs. We now know that it is this fat that causes problems, and this was the first clue to our understanding of why non-obese people can develop type 2 diabetes.

Insight from an Accident of Nature

Sometimes accidents of nature can propel a big jump forward in our scientific understanding. Some rare individuals, for example, are born with an absence of fat under the skin, and they survive by storing fat everywhere else. This condition is known as lipodystrophy and is caused by a single faulty gene. People with the condition look painfully thin, but their livers are full of fat. After reading Chapters 4 and 5, it may not surprise you to learn that they often have type 2 diabetes.

Holding up a mirror to today's population, anyone can see that the way fat is distributed on people's bodies varies hugely. Some people have big stomachs whereas others have large legs and buttocks. We now know, thanks to research carried out by a group of scientists at Cambridge University, that the maximum capacity of your own fat layer is determined by many genes, which each have a bearing; but that, apart from in rare conditions such as lipodystrophy, there is no single fat gene in the general population determining how much fat a person can store under the skin. Of course, how much you have stored under the skin also depends on how much you have eaten, and how much energy you have burned in daily activity—over a long period of time. We are very poor at conceptualizing time, whether it be geological time or the long periods over which tiny influences can produce major weight gain.

If, in the lottery that allocated your genes to you, your safe deposit for fat is rather limited, then you do not need to put on too much weight before fat has to build up elsewhere. And this, as we know from the Twin Cycle Hypothesis, is why some people will develop type 2 diabetes without being very heavy.

All of this can be distilled into one profoundly important fact: if an individual develops type 2 diabetes, they have become too heavy for their own body.

Too Heavy for Their Own Body

Samuel Johnson had a neat way with words and was a keen observer of people. Around 1790, he said: "If a man is too fat it is plain for all to see that he has eaten more than he should have done."

Note that he did not say that the person had "eaten too much." There was a subtlety that he recognized in implying that different individuals required different amounts of food. Now perhaps we can stand on the shoulders of giants and put together a succinct phrase about type 2 diabetes:

If a person has type 2 diabetes, they have become too heavy for their own body.

Testing the Hypothesis of a Personal Fat Threshold

The information from UKPDS was very helpful in supporting the Personal Fat Threshold concept. But it was another study—one not directed at type 2 diabetes—that provided crucial further substantiation.

The Nurses' Health Study is the world's largest, longest-running study of women's health. Set up in 1976 by a group of scientists at Harvard in the U.S., it has conducted a long-term follow-up of the impact of lifestyle factors on the health of some half a million young nurses—chosen, it should be said, not in order to study the risk factors of going into nursing as a career, but because nurses were thought likely to be able to provide accurate data.

With its regular follow-up of participants and repeated assessment of health and lifestyle factors, the study has played an instrumental role in shaping public health recommendations across the Western world. It helped uncover, for example, early links between cigarette smoking and both heart disease and cancer; between postmenopausal obesity and breast cancer; and has shed light on all sorts of other factors to do with health.

My interest was in weight gain, or rather in the fat threshold at which one woman versus another might develop type 2 diabetes. And what the study showed was this: those women who had stayed close to their youthful weight over several decades—i.e., remained with a BMI of under 22—were likely to have remained free of diabetes; but those who had increased their BMI even very slightly—to between 23 and 25—were much more likely to have developed the condition. This was no small increase in risk. The women whose weight had increased within the normal BMI range had a four times greater chance of developing type 2 diabetes compared to those whose BMI stayed less than 22.

To put this in context, big studies on large populations may show increased risk of, say, 15%. That often leads to exhortations to change your behavior or to avoid certain foods. It is said to be "statistically significant." But actually, an increased risk of 15% is only equivalent to a tiny change in your real risk. For instance, if you have a 1 in 10 chance of developing type 2 diabetes in the next 10 years and your risk increased by 15%, that would put your risk up to 1.15 in 10. Anyone familiar with betting odds might say, "So you are telling me that my risk changes from about 1 in 10 to about 1 in 10?" At the individual level it is not significant. On the other hand, the increase of four times means that your risk would rise to a 4 in 10 chance of getting type 2 diabetes, and for you that is a considerable increase in risk.

So, if these women who used to be young, healthy, and slim put on just a little weight, the level of risk of having type 2 diabetes increased considerably. Of course, if they put on even more weight, the risk went up much more. The study thus brilliantly shows how some individuals have a low threshold for tolerating excess fat.

We know that when a whole population becomes heavier, as is happening in many countries today, the overall effect is that the number of people developing type 2 diabetes increases. More people will have crossed their Personal Fat Threshold. Extrapolation of population trends to individuals has led to a widespread belief that a person's weight should be a good guide to whether or not they may have the disease. Having reached this point in the chapter you know that people of normal weight may develop type 2 diabetes.

Beware population statistics. Often-quoted figures on the risk of developing type 2 diabetes, such as "if BMI is greater than 30," are irrelevant to an individual who has developed the condition. We shall return to discuss risk factors in Chapter 9.

Susceptibility to Type 2 Diabetes

The Personal Fat Threshold explains why individuals may get type 2 diabetes at any level of BMI. But what does it look like if we examine the other half of the coin? How about very obese people who do not get type 2 diabetes?

In fact, the vast majority of very obese people do not have type 2 diabetes. The results of three large surveys throughout the U.S. showed that 72% of people with a BMI over 45 did not have diabetes. However, very obese people clearly have excess fat on board, and it is known that they tend to have fatty livers. Our recent research in the Magnetic Resonance Centre in Newcastle shows clearly that the excess fat does not produce type 2 diabetes in everyone. It merely sets in place the mechanism for excess fat to be produced by the liver and sent to the rest of the body, ensuring delivery of this potentially toxic stuff to the pancreas.

But there is a critical yes/no switch for diabetes.

Anyone developing type 2 diabetes is susceptible to the disease. That is obvious. Also, they must have beta cells that are susceptible to the adverse effects of fat. But not everyone has this susceptibility. For a long time, we have known that most human genes linked to type 2 diabetes are something to do with the pancreas. Now we have a big clue that at least some of them determine whether you will or will not get diabetes if too much fat builds up there.

Looking Inside the Beta Cell

Back in the early 1990s, Roger Unger, one of the brilliant minds of diabetes, did a study involving rats that demonstrated that susceptibility to fat in the beta cells came down to a single defective gene. That gene determined whether or not an animal would develop type 2 diabetes when overfed.

Unger and his team took beta cells from young rats with the diabetes gene well before diabetes had developed and incubated the cells with fat for several days. What Unger and his team found was that the fat impaired the cells' ability to make insulin in response to an increase in glucose. That was interesting in itself.

They then ran the same experiment on rats that were similar in all respects except that they did not have the gene defect that conferred susceptibility to diabetes. Beta cells from these rats tested with fat exposure carried on making insulin normally. The excess fat had no effect, proving that the ultimate susceptibility to diabetes lay in the beta cells themselves.

The full implications of Unger's work have lain dormant for almost three decades. Knowing about the Personal Fat Threshold in humans, we can now see that, in a stroke of brilliance, he had laid the groundwork for understanding why obese people did not usually get type 2 diabetes. The single major gene defect in unusual rats showed a basic biological mechanism. Detailed genetic studies in humans have shown that there is no one gene for susceptibility to type 2 diabetes, and it is almost certain that susceptibility must be determined by a number of genes, each contributing a little. Just like the story of the lipodystrophy gene, which led the way to the demonstration of the genetic basis determining the safe maximum storage capacity of the fat layer under the skin, it helped us understand how different combinations of many weaker genes will determine how susceptible your beta cells are to fat accumulation.

Armed with this insight, scientists can now ask focused questions. Which human genes contribute most to susceptibility to the toxic effect of fat? How do they interact? Are there separate genes determining whether beta cells remain able to recover even after decades of suppression by fat?

Your eclectic collection of genes determines the degree of fat exposure at which your beta cells will stop responding to glucose. If you have developed diabetes, you have beta cells that are susceptible to fat-induced damage. But the good news is: no fat, no damage.

Quick Read

- Type 2 diabetes is not caused by obesity
- Everyone has a Personal Fat Threshold above which they might develop type 2 diabetes
- This is determined initially by a number of genes that dictate how much fat can be stored safely—under the skin

- Above the Personal Fat Threshold, excess fat will be supplied by the liver to all tissues of the body, including the pancreas
- Even if you exceed your Personal Fat Threshold, though, the stop/go determinant for type 2 is inside your beta cells: they may or may not be susceptible to the bad effects of excess fat
- Even if you are doubly unlucky and have both a limited capacity to store fat under the skin and fat-susceptible beta cells: no excess fat, no diabetes

7

Escaping from Type 2 Diabetes

Okay, time for action. Having gained an understanding of how the body works and why diabetes occurs, we can now look at how to get rid of it. In this chapter, I outline the "1,2,3" approach, originally designed to identify the cause of type 2 diabetes but found to be successful in real life. This is a simple program, with clearly defined stages—first, lose weight rapidly with a clear end point; second, reintroduce ordinary foods step by step; third, keep the weight down long term.

A rapid weight loss phase followed by a stepped return to normal eating is very different from the standard advice of "slow and prolonged" of recent years. The 1,2,3 approach recognizes that losing weight is a distinct activity, separate from the matter of keeping the weight steady in the long term, and that there are many benefits from losing weight fast in the first instance. There are other approaches to losing weight. However, several high-quality studies have shown that going on an intensive rapid weight loss diet for a period is not only effective for most people but extraordinarily motivating.

How to Do It

1. **Recognize the problem:**
   If you have type 2 diabetes you have become too heavy for your body
2. **Write down your target weight:**
   Usually a weight loss of around 33 pounds
3. **Recognize that food intake has to be decreased for 2–3 months:**
   Think when it may suit you to do this
4. **Discuss with family and friends:**
   Support is one of the secrets of success
5. **Decide:**
   Do you really want to do this?
6. **Prepare for action:**
   Clear the cupboards
7. **Action:**
   Do it

1. Recognize the Problem

For centuries, type 2 diabetes has been thought of as a lifelong condition. The data from the famous United Kingdom Prospective Diabetes Study (UKPDS) "proved" this, didn't it? In that study, folks had to take more and more tablets year by year, yet their blood sugar control continued to deteriorate. There appeared to be an inevitable downhill path, whether sugar levels were initially kept as low as possible or not so low. After 10 years of this grim progression, as many as half of the people in the study needed insulin injections.

So why did that study prove that type 2 diabetes always progressed and never went away? The simple answer is that people in this study did not lose weight. In fact, the reverse happened. This is the case in real life too: despite being advised to lose some weight, people recently diagnosed with type 2 diabetes find that their weight creeps up over ensuing years. This may not surprise those who have been on the receiving end of routine advice about weight loss. It is often handed out with no conviction that it is possible, and without specific instructions on how to do it. Even if guideline-based advice from a dietitian is available, this is often frustratingly ineffective. Most people's steady increase in weight after being diagnosed with type 2 does not surprise doctors either, as they know that some of the tablets prescribed to manage the condition actually hamper weight loss.

In the bodies of those people who took part in the UKPDS study, the levels of fat inside the liver and pancreas must have remained high. Tablets will have improved their blood glucose levels but this is not relevant for the progression of the disease. Inside the pancreas, the insulin-producing beta cells were slowly being inactivated and consequently all hope of adequate blood glucose control slowly faded.

But the information from UKPDS could not be properly understood, as the precise cause of type 2 diabetes was still unknown. Now that we do know it, the real message from the study can be seen from a whole new perspective.

If body weight stays as high as it has become by the time type 2 diabetes is diagnosed—then the diabetes does not go away and will get worse. If you lose a lot of weight, though, the very opposite is true.

Your type 2 diabetes has been caused by less than half a gram of fat inside your pancreas. That small amount of excess fat is inside the cells, preventing the proper manufacture and release of insulin. There is not only excess fat within the cells of the pancreas, but too much in the blood, continuously arriving and adding to the burden. Is there not some clever way of getting rid of this small amount of fat that is in the wrong place?

Sadly not. The only way of decreasing this burden of fat is to decrease the total amount of fat accumulated in your body—not just by a few pounds, but by a lot. Once this is crystal clear, escape from type 2 diabetes is within your grasp. You need to lose weight and keep it off.

2. Write Down Your Target Weight

However much fat you may have in your body, the development of type 2 diabetes is telling you that you have too much. Too much for your personal constitution. Don't compare your size with that of others. You are yourself. Your constitution is different from that of others. The purpose of the section on the Personal Fat Threshold in Chapter 6 was to explain that if you have type 2 diabetes, your body is simply telling you that it has too much fat on board.

How much is too much fat?

As a rule of thumb, decreasing your body weight by 33 pounds will correct the excess of fat. It is the same whether you weigh 176 pounds or 352 pounds, as this is highly likely to take you below your Personal Fat Threshold (but see the chart on page 162). Losing so much weight may sound like an impossible task, but it is easier than you may think. The method devised to test the Twin Cycle Hypothesis—cutting calorie intake to around 700 calories daily—was found to be surprisingly straightforward by the pioneers who volunteered for the Counterpoint study. It was certainly not easy—but far less difficult than any of them expected. What helps is that the average weight loss after one week is around 8 pounds—and this makes a profound difference to how people feel day to day. Just try to get up out of a chair or walk upstairs while carrying this weight, say, as a bag of potatoes. Then do the same without. All daily activities suddenly become very much easier when you are lighter. You will soon feel so much better that your motivation will be reinforced.

Yes, you will feel very hungry for the first 36 hours, but hardly at all after that. The ongoing problems are more about adjusting daily life around some major changes. Perhaps not joining in with family mealtimes or other social eating. Perhaps doing business without a business lunch. Perhaps ensuring that if you are out and about you have come prepared and will not end up being tempted to buy something on the hoof. Compared with the miserable and often ineffective rigmarole of trying to lose weight over six months or a year, losing substantial amounts of weight rapidly is so much easier.

So, if you weigh 176 pounds, weight loss of about 33–55 pounds is likely to return glucose control to normal—provided you have not had type 2 diabetes for too long. The only way to know whether your diabetes has gone too far to be reversed is to lose the weight and see. As mentioned above, there are individuals with long-duration diabetes who have successfully escaped.

It is worth repeating that the aim is not the usual, unfocused one of becoming non-obese. Obesity itself is not relevant. What is important is to get yourself below your Personal Fat Threshold. And 33 pounds is the magic number to lose whether you start at 352 pounds or 176 pounds. Of course, there may be other health gains to be had from losing even more weight, but this book is about returning to metabolic health, not becoming slim.

The 33 pounds rule of thumb works fine for most people but may be too much if you are not a big person. You can still be above your Personal Fat Threshold yet not heavy—compared with others. At a lower starting weight, say, below 176 pounds, it is better to think about losing 15% of your body weight. So Mrs. One Hundred and Thirty-Two Pounds could reasonably aim to lose 20 pounds.

The first step is to look at the chart on the next page and write down your target weight. Don't be put off by the seeming difficulty—hundreds of people like you have achieved similar weight loss. It can be done. Just like moving to the long-term home of your dreams, you should start looking forward to it. Write it down. Then it is a real target.

If your current weight in pounds is:	Then your target weight might be:
330	297
325	292
320 315 310 305	287 282 277 272
300	267
295	262
290	257
285	252
280	247
275 270	242 237
265	232
260	227
255	222
250	217
245	212
240	207

7.1 For anyone with type 2 diabetes who is considering trying to escape from the condition, this chart shows approximately which weight they should be aiming for. Don't be daunted by the challenge.

3. Recognize That Food Intake Has to Be Decreased for 2–3 Months

When will you start on your escape diet? Certainly not instantaneously—as you need to plan ahead. Perhaps after the family party next week? This is not an invitation to put it off, then put it off again, but rather to encourage you to take a cool look ahead to check that you are making things as easy as possible for yourself. Choose your time.

Many people struggle to find two to three months when there are no social occasions, upheavals at work, holidays etc. So plans need to be laid for how you will manage to stay on course. If you have a party or event, you could opt to take your own food or shake. Perhaps make sure you drink only water or zero-calorie beverages? Leave before the food is served? Some people have told me that they tended to eat their special meals before going out to the event as they tend to be very filling. Then they wouldn't let a morsel pass their lips during the event. Enlisting support from everyone close to you will be extremely helpful.

There is always, of course, the option of taking a break from your diet for, say, a special weekend. But you have to bear in mind that this is the more difficult option, not least because that brief diet holiday will be followed by a further 36 hours of feeling hungry again as your body reacclimatizes. In my view, breaks should be the exception, reserved for only very special occasions. Otherwise, there is a risk that they become the norm and overeating starts to creep back in, hampering your escape effort. The decision has to be yours. But remember that learning how to manage social occasions involving food and drink is a valuable skill for future maintenance and will stand you in good stead forever.

4. Discuss with Friends and Family

I can't stress this point enough. Obviously, it is important to enlist the support of family and friends to help during all the difficulties that crop up as part of life. But contemplating major weight loss is a far more pervasive thing. Eating is a social activity, and usually involves your nearest and dearest. Just consider meeting a friend. How often would you drink or eat with them, just as an accepted part of the occasion? Many families eat together as a routine. Therefore, any change you make to what and how much you eat will impinge upon everyone else in the house. If the whole family is willing to make some changes at the same time, this may ease some of the difficulties. Similarly, with friends and workmates. You need allies.

What does your spouse/partner/close friend think about you embarking on this challenge to get rid of your diabetes? Will they be happy or less than happy to see you at a lighter weight and feeling 10 years younger? Maybe there might even be a message in all this for them? What do they think of the information that they themselves are on average 22 pounds heavier than their alter ego would have been in 1980? In our early studies, only three people dropped out, and in all these cases the reason was that their spouse/

partner did not want them to lose more weight. That may appear surprising, but perceptions vary. And philosophers tell us that perceptions are the only reality—in other words, not everyone sees you in the same light.

A family resolve to avoid eating anything other than at mealtimes is a clear-cut first step. In today's overfed society, snacking between meals has become the norm; we are tempted at every turn by biscuits and cakes and sugary drinks. But just 50 years ago, this sort of overfeeding would have seemed absurd. We are now frequently unable to tell the difference between boredom and real hunger. Often the phrase "I feel a bit peckish" really means "nothing much doing just now." Spot the difference. But if something has to go constantly from hand to mouth, perhaps water will do.

If there are no biscuits, crisps, or sweets in the cupboards, moments of temptation are much easier to deal with. There is much talk these days about the "obesogenic environment" in which we live—our sedentary lifestyle, our use of cars and labor-saving machines, and our ready access to fast foods. However, the obesogenic microenvironment of the home is easily overlooked. That microenvironment can be changed if the family is willing. Many of our research volunteers have described such a revolution.

Beware the excuses you may make to yourself and others, for example: "I need to keep some treats in the cupboards for the children/grandchildren." First, remember that type 2 diabetes runs in families, and families will share the genes that determine the risk for type 2 diabetes. So setting up your youngsters to have treats as a routine will do them no favors in the long term. Far better would be to actively help them avoid having to make the same escape effort that you are contemplating just now. Second, if you are tempted to eat the treats, then they were probably never really for the grandchildren anyway. Being honest with yourself in this regard is hard at first, but important. If you are unable to resist them, they will have to go.

5. Decide

How do you make a decision? Some people weigh up all the facts, ponder on them for a while, and only then come to a conclusion. Other people—maybe a majority—come to a snap decision either immediately on hearing the pros and cons or later triggered by something else.

Psychologists used to talk about something called "the cycle of change." This was the idea that everyone went first through a phase of pre-contemplation, not yet thinking about any decision, then a phase of contemplation, weighing up advantages and disadvantages. Next there would be preparation, the intention to make a decision, and then, finally, a phase of action. It is now recognized that most people do not go through these theoretical stages but rather come to a rapid decision at an unpredictable time. This decision may be precipitated by events or ideas that may seem to you completely unrelated and which you don't recognize as the trigger for moving your mind forward.

Imagine, if instead of diabetes, you had developed a life-threatening disease that could only be cured by an operation, and that your doctor said to you that this would mean taking three months off work, and stopping all normal activities of life. Faced with a life-threatening condition, you would not hesitate to accept this. It would be a no-brainer. You would plan for the operation and work out how to fit your life around this period of downtime.

Given that type 2 diabetes causes all the misery and shortening of life described in Chapter 1, the same thinking should be applied. It is a serious condition that threatens your eyesight, your feet, and your heart, not to mention doubling the risk of a stroke at any age. There are other repercussions too. You have acquired a disease label. Unthinkingly, people now refer to you as "a diabetic"; you find yourself sitting for long periods in clinic waiting rooms; your holiday insurance costs twice as much; you face a lifetime of monitoring and medication.

With the 1,2,3 approach, your route to fixing this is much less disruptive than taking, say, three months off work for surgery. During your period of low-calorie dieting, work and everyday life will continue. You may worry that you won't have enough energy to do your usual work, but do not fear—most people report feeling more energetic than usual while dieting. This may be contrary to what you would expect, but in our experience with the volunteers for the DiRECT study, most felt better than before and the few who did feel a bit tired (one in 15) were still able to continue at work, as the potential prize at the end kept them motivated and made their efforts feel worthwhile.

I could come up with any number of reasons to try to convince you that embarking on this program is a good idea. But it is of course a challenge, and some people may feel that they would prefer just to take the pills and accept whatever fate has in store for them. It has to be a personal choice. But in my experience many folk would really like their health back—as soon as possible. Health is one of those things that never seem precious until they been lost.

Don't forget the previous point. Do talk it over with your spouse, partner, family, or friends. Ideally, everyone will get behind your mission, if not actively involved in it. Others will be affected by your decision.

But whatever the process for you, and however wide-ranging the discussion, a decision needs to be taken. You will know when you have decided. And provided you have been given the information about the alternatives, no one can tell you that your decision is wrong or right—it is *your* decision.

Don't rush through this step. Just be sure that you are sure.

6. Prepare for Action

Check those cupboards. Are they clear of biscuits, cakes, and chips? Do you have all the supplies you need? Packets to make up liquid meals? Salad stuffs and other non-starchy veg? A glass at the ready for water? If you work away from home, it would be a good idea to stock up on packed-lunch equipment—Tupperware for salads, thermal mugs for soup—so you can be forearmed. It is essential to plan ahead so you don't get done in by hunger pangs and end up buying a snack that is bulging with calories.

Are your supporters ready and tuned into your plans?

One curious thing must be considered. You may have friends, relatives, or acquaintances who do not seem to want you to lose weight and may actively engage in what could be called sabotage. "You will have a muffin, won't you?" This can be particularly difficult to deal with when you are trying to keep to a strict regime. It is a good idea to think through how you might respond to this sort of thing before you start.

7. Action!

All our research work on reversing type 2 diabetes has depended upon a method for losing weight that can be achieved by all the participants within a defined period of time—a combination of low-calorie soups and shakes to maintain a daily intake around the 800-calorie mark (in our Counterpoint study, we got our volunteers to stick to around 700 calories per day for 8 weeks, but in DiRECT around 800 for 12 weeks). In a research study, it is vital to have a uniform, reproducible way of bringing about change that is acceptable to most people. But you are not most people. You are an individual and, for a range of reasons, you may be able to achieve the goal—33-pound weight loss—by other means. Perhaps you hate the idea of low-calorie drinks and would rather cook for yourself. And that is fine. Whatever works for you.

You need to plan for long-term weight control right from the beginning. And then, once you have shed the 33 pounds, and after you have congratulated yourself (and your supporters), you need to be prepared for the fact that you will need less food than you previously ate. In practice, this will be around three quarters of the amount you habitually put on your plate and swallowed. Remember, this marks the beginning of the rest of your life. And eating less will be the only way to maintain your new, healthy, comparatively svelte form. Knowing this from the outset is important.

The 1,2,3 Approach

In our early studies in Newcastle to test the Twin Cycle Hypothesis, we had to come up with a simple, practical, and effective way for our volunteers to achieve a big change in body weight. In the first instance, I devised an eight-week program of low-calorie powdered shakes, offering complete nutrition in an easy way, requiring minimum prep. Complete nutrition means that the diet provided all the necessary protein, minerals, and micronutrients. More fiber was provided by a daily helping of non-starchy vegetables. Following the first trial, however, our research volunteers told us of the difficulty they had had in restarting normal eating. They described how, after eight weeks of simply choosing which flavor packet to make up in water, they were all at sea, or even panicky, when trying to prepare a meal. As a result, we devised a clearly directed stepped approach, whereby first one meal of normal foodstuffs (usually the evening meal) was substituted for a shake for at least two weeks, and then, a week later, the same was done for lunch. If the individual was ready, breakfast could then be restarted. The quantity of food was carefully described—usually about three quarters of that habitually eaten before weight loss.

We used this stepped food reintroduction in the Counterbalance study and were pleased to find that the participants avoided the problems of a sudden switch—and could keep their weight steady after rapid weight loss. The low-calorie weight loss phase followed by the new stepped program became known as the Newcastle Diet. And then, for the DiRECT study, we used a similar strategy that had been separately developed in Glasgow as Counterweight-Plus.

First get the weight down, focusing entirely on that. Second, reintroduce ordinary foods step by step. Then third, keep the weight down long term.

Recognizing that these stages are three clear-cut operations is important. Careful research has shown that major weight loss can be achieved by this clear separation of a relatively short but intense period of weight loss from the long-term keep-it-down phase. But a word of caution is needed: the best studies to date have lasted for only two years, and weight regain must be avoided for life. Phase 3 is the most challenging. (Further information is available on the website: https://go.ncl.ac.uk/diabetes-reversal.)

What to Eat: Overview

Step 1. For the 8 weeks of rapid weight loss, the simplest option is to use a liquid formula product to provide around 600 calories per day, with one helping of non-starchy vegetables (around 100 calories). No alcohol (and no additional exercise).

Step 2. For the transition to normal eating, one small meal of ordinary foods (of 400–500 calories) is substituted for the evening liquid meal for approximately 2 weeks. Then a small lunch (around 400 calories) is introduced for the next 2 weeks. Then the liquid meals are stopped.

Step 3. For long-term weight maintenance, your weighing scales are your best friend. Eating is back to being a normal, social activity—but with a close eye on quantities. The same goes for alcohol.

Food vs. Liquid Formula

Having a packet of one of the many commercially available liquid formula diets per meal is by far the easier option for most people. Some brands have a wide range of flavors to choose from and minimize boredom. On our

Newcastle Diet, we also encouraged participants to add in some non-starchy veg at mealtimes, partly for something to chew on (an activity that is badly missed by some) but mainly because veg help to avoid constipation. (In our DiRECT trial we missed out the vegetables in favor of a fourth packet of liquid formula meal because of the need to minimize differences between people in this research study; however, regular laxatives were needed with this regime to deal with constipation.)

And, if you can't bear the idea of going on liquid formula drinks for several weeks with or without vegetables, you can of course use ordinary foods. You would have to make up meals containing around 200 calories, with no more than 800 calories a day. This involves a lot of planning and preparation time in the kitchen, and many people find it more difficult because of the daily burden of decisions and choices.

If you go for real foods to provide approximately 800 calories per day, you would need a high proportion of protein foods (fish, meat) both to meet your daily need for protein and to keep you satisfied for longer. Plenty of non-starchy vegetables are important to fill you up and keep your bowels regular. It may take you a bit longer to cruise down to your target weight—about three to four months as opposed to two to three months on the liquid formula.

There is also a possibility that you could run a little short on some vitamins, and for this reason food-based diets of around 800 calories per day are best supplemented with a multivitamin tablet.

Step 1 in Practice

Choose your low-calorie diet. If it is to be a liquid diet, then you must decide which brand and which flavors you like. Whichever brand you choose, it *must* be described as "complete nutrition" (as opposed to just a "meal replacement")—in other words, that it contains all the vitamins, minerals, and trace elements in addition to protein, sugar, and fat.

You may be surprised by the high sugar content of some brands—but don't worry as this is low compared with what your liver makes every day. The protein content will be high: around 25% and much higher than you might usually eat in a meal. It must come as one packet per meal (no decisions or room for inadvertently adjusted doses). Each packet will contain around 200 calories (see our website for a list of suitable products: https://go.ncl.ac.uk/diabetes-reversal).

Liquid diets are easier for most people, and bear in mind that this is what was used in the research that showed major weight loss and lasting remission of type 2 diabetes. To maintain an adequate intake of fiber, you have the option of either taking a fiber supplement, or eating a single helping of non-starchy vegetables each day, in addition to your shakes. (See the recipe section.)

If you are going for the real-food option, or even a mixture of the two, you will need to be well prepared with the right ingredients and recipes to keep you going. And be realistic: you will not want to spend hours preparing gourmet low-calorie meals every day; have some quick, easy, calorie-counted options at the ready—some grilled chicken or fish with a pile of non-starchy vegetables, for example. Make this your default main meal every day if need be.

Do not embark on an exercise program during Step 1. Perhaps surprisingly, this can seriously impede weight loss especially in very overweight people. This may be the best-kept secret in the weight loss field, and I came across it only from listening to participants in one of our exercise studies. They described "compensatory eating" (part conscious and part-subconscious). So just remain normally active during Step 1.

- Write down why you are doing this. This can be really useful to read later if you are struggling with the balance between daily life and avoiding putting weight back on.
- During a liquid diet, you will have lots of time on your hands as you won't be preparing food and perhaps won't even be sitting at the family table at mealtimes, so plan ahead as to what you are going to do with that time. Write a list.
- Then plan what you are going to do if you feel tempted to eat something off-limits. Writing your own list of distractions can be helpful—jobs around the house, surprising the dog with an extra walk, drinking a pint of water, planning future holidays.

- You also need to plan for how to supply yourself with your special meals when out of the house. This is easiest if your chosen liquid diet powder is designed to be dissolved in water rather than milk, but advance planning will make things manageable in either case.
- No alcohol during the weight loss phase. Alcohol is high in calories. Think of it as liquid fat. Not helpful. Just don't do it.
- Continue to enjoy tea and coffee, with skimmed milk if preferred (not more than 2 ounces per day).
- Discuss your plans with your doctor or diabetes nurse.

This is what people said about their experience of the liquid diet in our studies:

> *"I was so surprised, what I was eating compared to what I have been eating over the last weeks I really would have thought that I would have been hungry from the moment I opened my eyes to the moment I closed my eyes, but I wasn't." (Woman, aged 42, one year after reversing to normal.)*

> *"It was fairly hard to start with but it got easier as the weeks went on and then when I started getting*

a bit fitter and could walk further and stand up and sit down and dig the garden it's great now. I feel great." (Man, aged 44, two and a half years since diagnosis.)

Although the majority reflected these thoughts, not everyone found it feasible:

"Because the smells of people eating all around you . . . I was in town at one point, bakeries everywhere and, it was ridiculous, I couldn't concentrate . . . would have been fine if I had been at home. I would have lost weight this week and I would have still been on it, but I couldn't stick to it." (Man, aged 52, one year since diagnosis.)

The next quote gives an insight into what has happened to our main streets and elsewhere over the last two to three decades. This person was not alone in lamenting the all-pervasive offerings of food in our society today:

"You just can't get away from food. Pick up the paper and there is Jamie Oliver doing something clever with a leg of lamb. Turn on the telly and there is Mary Berry baking cakes. So you take yourself off to the football only to find yourself surrounded by hamburger adverts and stalls. I couldn't sit at the family dinner table. I had to fill in time by going to the cinema to watch just anything. Poor sad old

geezer sitting by himself. But it worked." (Man, aged 57, still free of diabetes two years after the study.)

Step 2 in Practice

Moving from the weight loss phase back to eating ordinary foods needs some careful planning. We realized this after the Counterpoint study, which was designed only to test the Twin Cycle Hypothesis. We had focused mainly on how to lose a lot of weight fast, without sufficiently thinking through the challenge of the re-entry period. Our research volunteers described feeling all at sea on going back into the kitchen. What to eat? How much to eat? Could they drink?

But what we also learned was that there was an opportunity for people here: eight weeks of just eating a packet for each meal created a blank slate on which to write new dietary habits.

Just as there is a clear focus during the initial weight loss phase, there must also be a definite plan for the stepped food reintroduction phase.

- Start with the evening meal, going back to eating a normal (but smaller than usual) plate of food instead of the shake, but continuing your weight loss diet during the rest of the day.
- It is sensible to do some advance planning here too: a normal meal should still be

relatively low in carbohydrates and contain plenty of veg. Avoid sweet or starchy foods.

- After two weeks, you can add in a lunchtime meal, stopping the shake but, again, exercising portion control.
- After four weeks, you can be back into a fairly normal pattern of eating that is sustainable for life—without regaining weight. And drink alcohol if you wish. It is normal during this phase for your weight to rise by around 2 pounds because glycogen stores are building back up—and water is always stored along with glycogen.

Using stepped food reintroduction, our volunteers found the transition to normal eating to be less troublesome and more sustainable in the long term. They reported that the directed approach to starting one low-calorie meal per day was helpful. They also appreciated being armed with definitive information about what quantity of which food to eat. More information about foods for this stage is given in the recipe section at the back.

Step 3 in Practice

By this stage you should feel very proud of yourself. You will have lost a substantial amount of weight; you will hopefully have achieved remission of your type 2 diabetes; and you will be feeling dramatically better, both in mind and body: more energized, confident, and motivated. Welcome to the beginning of your new life.

Perhaps it would be safer to call it the "new normal." It is so worthwhile to work at maintaining your newly recovered health. While you can enjoy eating with family and friends again, and even indulge in a special treat or the occasional party, if you want to keep the weight off you simply must avoid slipping back into your old ways and habits.

Stick with these rules of thumb and you will be fine:

- As a rough guide, you will need to eat only three quarters of the amount that you used to eat.
- Write down your weight each week. This is essential. Your weighing scales will tell it how it is. Day to day, your weight may fluctuate, but week to week if you see steadily rising numbers you are eating—or maybe drinking—too much. Figure out the best way for you to consume less food or alcohol. Be more active each day. This has to be built into the routine of life and not something that requires a decision. Get into the habit of walking rather than driving. Always take the stairs. Are there any particular activities that would encourage you to be active for longer, most days? If it is your thing, go dancing or get back to badminton. Is there a local 5-a-side

league? Remember, the best form of exercise is the one that you enjoy.

- If your weight rises by 7 pounds above target, take immediate action. Recognize the writing on the wall without delay. You need either to go back to the liquid formula diet for a few weeks or drastically decrease your daily amount of food. Ask yourself whether your alcohol intake is the problem. Whatever you do, don't abandon all your hard work in regaining health. Think back to why you took action in the first place. In DiRECT, such rescue plans were needed by one person in two. Weight regain is not necessarily failure. Life will have its ups and downs. But you do not have to be a casualty. Make sure it is only a temporary blip.
- Beware of activities that often involve communal snacking such as watching television. Don't snack—drink water. Or sit on your hands. Ideally, the intensive period of dieting will have changed some of your habits. Certainly, it is best to avoid any pastime in which hands are apt to move subconsciously and continuously between packet and mouth.
- Take pride in your written record of weekly weight so that you can say: "I'm the same

weight as I was at the age of [25?] and have been for a year." And the last couple of words will eventually become five years . . . 10 years . . . 20 years.

- And, finally, ensure that life is enjoyable. Yes, total calories need to be limited to whatever level allows your weight to stay steady, but this should not become a daily burden. It is not the one-off blow-out, but the everyday, background intake of calories that is determinant.

So party, but pay back. You can now join in celebrating the way-markers of life—anniversaries, birthdays, family occasions—indeed you must! But then you must recognise the need to eat less during the following week. How will you do this? Perhaps by having half-sized portions at one meal each day for the week, or, if intermittent fasting suits you, one day of eating very little. Once again, you need to have a definitive plan ready to put into action.

Of course, all this is easier to describe than to achieve, and you are bound to come up against tricky moments. Descriptions of the challenges faced by our volunteers during the weight maintenance phase were gathered during the psychological research conducted as part of Counterbalance. They reflect real-life events like this one:

> *"I was so frazzled I went up to the desk and there was some chocolates right in front of us [me] and I was so tempted to have one but I walked away*

from them, although I have to say I walked up to the tin and lifted the lid three times but each time I just walked away from it because I thought no, because that would have felt like I had given in and I didn't want to do that." (Woman, aged 35, one and a half years since diagnosis.)

Why Might Previous Weight Loss Attempts Have Failed?

In the Counterbalance and DiRECT studies, a team of psychologists led by Professor Falko Sniehotta interviewed the participants to find out what had contributed to their success in keeping their weight steady, and also what had been the main barriers to success. Prior to joining the study, many participants had tried and failed to lose weight and keep it off. One of the main reasons for this was the slow rate of their weight loss; over a prolonged period of trying to adhere to a regime boredom had set in. Or social habits around food were difficult to change. On their previous diets, some people had experienced nagging hunger, and had actively disliked the extent of the food restriction necessary to continue losing weight. By contrast, most participants viewed the 1,2,3 approach favorably in general, both for its speed and because they had felt so well during the low-calorie phase. They also said that ongoing support from their general-practice nurse or dietitian was useful in prompting action if their weight started to edge upward.

The longer follow-up, still ongoing in DiRECT, is showing us that weight regain remains a challenge. There are no easy answers. The general advice above is the best we can do at present. Stick with it!

Why Lose Weight Rapidly?

If food intake is decreased to around 800 calories per day for a two-month period, there are several advantages. Once underway, you are unlikely to feel very hungry. This is possibly a survival mechanism that evolved during our hunter-gatherer millennia. It would have been difficult to hunt successfully if all you could think about was being ravenously hungry. A second major advantage is that you start feeling so much better within a short period of time that you will want to keep going. You'll find you move around more easily; you sleep much more soundly. You will start feeling more energetic.

In the first week of a 700–800 calorie diet, the average weight loss is 8 pounds. During the whole eight weeks it is just over 33 pounds. This might sound rather alarming: is it healthy to cut back so much on eating? Sudden weight loss is usually thought of as an indicator of serious disease. But the hard evidence is that for anyone who has increased their weight during adult life, or has always been overweight, losing the extra weight and then eating less long term is of huge benefit to health. In our overfed society, fasting is not usually dangerous, but eating is.

As I mentioned above, if you opt for total food replacement using a liquid product to lose weight, there are some additional advantages. The first is that it is easy to have a high proportion of protein at each meal, and this helps to control hunger. The second is that there are no difficult choices about what and how much to eat. Freeing yourself from the cumulative burden of decisions, decisions, decisions makes weight loss genuinely easier.

You don't have to lose weight fast to reverse your diabetes, but for most people it's the easiest way of losing the requisite number of pounds. Overall, the 1,2,3 approach works because the defined goals of each stage are humanly possible, and the early wins increase motivation to succeed.

Strategies for Behavior Regulation

A lot of what we do from day to day is subconscious. Our actions are determined to a large extent by habit and social conformity, and it is worth trying to identify particular influences that might be modifiable. In Newcastle, Professor Sniehotta and his team have identified some potentially useful strategies to consider:

- Avoidance. Identify situations of maximum pressure to conform with social eating.
- Distraction. Have your own list of things that you need to do. Mending, fixing, phoning—all the things that may be difficult

to pull to mind at the critical moment, but can be remembered and listed from time to time. Add to the to-do list: "Write to MP to remind him/her of the importance of legislation to restrain commercially driven excess calorie provision."

- Drinking water. Tap water is inexpensive. Keep a large jug in the fridge. Drinking a pint of water fills the stomach and also occupies the mind during moments of temptation. Have fizzy water for a change. Flavored waters with zero calories are also an option to have in the fridge.
- Removing the wrong sort of food from your environment. Your cupboards will ideally be a biscuit-, chip-, cake-, and chocolate-free zone.
- Reminding yourself of your goals. Write down why you wanted to escape from diabetes in the first place. This can be just a few words on the first page of your diary or on your phone. Read it every now and then. The reasons why you started out on this program tend to blur and fade with time: 1. Wanting not to suffer like Dad; 2. Wanting not to have the tummy upset from those tablets; 3. Wanting not to worry about eyesight or feet or heart; 4. Feeling generally unhealthy. Your reasons will be

just as valid years later—if only you could remember them.

- Social disclosure. Your family will already be well aware of why they should not offer you biscuits with your coffee. Hopefully, you can also be entirely open with colleagues and friends about your aim to stay healthy by minimizing the chronic food poisoning. It is true, not everyone is as susceptible to this food poisoning as you have found out that you are. Your explanations should not be seen as preaching to all—but everyone can benefit from knowing that body weight should not rise during adult life.

Frequently Asked Questions

Is the speed of weight loss important?

It is important only in that fast weight loss makes losing 33 pounds easier for most people. The effect of removing fat from the liver and then the pancreas is the same whether weight loss happens over two months or a year. The simple biology of type 2 diabetes speaks for itself: get the excess fat out of the pancreas and the insulin production starts up again (as long as the beta cells have not been damaged for too long).

I have been told I have pre-diabetes. What should I do?

Get started on the 1,2,3. By losing approximately 22 pounds (or 10% of your weight if you are less than 176 pounds) you will almost certainly take yourself out of this category and transform your chances of remaining healthy long term.

Can I use a milk diet?

Ideally, you will use the liquid formula packets that provide complete nutrition. But if there is some reason why this is not feasible, then yes, a milk-based diet (2 liters of semi-skimmed milk per day) is both inexpensive and feasible. It will be important to take a multivitamin tablet daily and to eat some non-starchy vegetables—to provide some roughage and something to chew on.

Can I really not drink alcohol during Step 1?

No, because alcohol is effectively liquid fat, as explained in Chapter 2. Alcoholic drinks contain far more calories than is generally realized. It is easier for most people to completely cut out all alcohol-containing drinks during Step 1. However, one of our most successful research participants insisted on having a glass of red wine every Friday evening. It was sipped very slowly and not refilled.

The acid test is whether you are achieving adequate weight loss. So, provided that you lose around 8 pounds in the first week and around 3 pounds each week after that, a glass of wine per week may be fine. Beer would be problematic, given that it is so full of calories (around 200 in one pint!).

Why do I feel cold?

Some people do feel cold all the time while losing weight. A common misconception is that this is due to the thinning of the insulating layer of fat under the skin—a most unlikely explanation since coldness tends to come on so soon after starting to lose weight. Feeling cold is more likely to be caused by the smaller amounts of heat generated by the body when deprived of calories. The only thing you can do is wrap up warmly (thermal vest?) and accept it as a better option than being too heavy and too sweaty.

Will my thinning hair regrow?

This is unusual, but the answer is yes—providing that it is due to the sudden change in nutrition. A few people notice hair loss after weight loss. In fact, under any unusual circumstance (exams, pregnancy, family illness) the growth cycle of hair follicles tends to become synchronized, which means that instead of losing the normal 70 hairs per day as they come to the end of their growth cycle and fall out, several hundred fall out every day for a short time. But don't worry—they will all grow back over a few months.

How can I fix my constipation?

There are people who, despite chomping through a large plate of lettuce, celery, peppers, and tomatoes every single day, find that they are still constipated while dieting. What to do? The simplest thing is to ask your own doctor to prescribe a medicine that will bulk up your bowel movements.

Can weight loss cause gallstones?

A low-calorie diet generally makes gallstones smaller, which means there is a small chance that they may squeeze into the biliary duct (through which the digestive juices enter the gut), causing pain. Among people with type 2 diabetes, gallstones are very common—they are present in around one person in five. In our DiRECT trial, only one person of the 149 undergoing weight loss had gall bladder trouble during the study. This is not very different from the number that would be expected in a group of people with type 2 diabetes undergoing standard medical treatment. Therefore, although there is a small risk of having a biliary attack as gallstones get smaller, if no weight is lost there is a greater chance of a future episode of gallstone pain anyway.

Can I change where the fat disappears from?

Sometimes it seems as though the fat is dropping away, but from all the wrong places. Sadly, we have no way of affecting this. In fact, it is amazing that even now, with our detailed knowledge about so much of the human body, we have no idea why fat is stored in the places it is on any one person's body. What controls this? What stops it being heaped together in a hump somewhere? Bar the obvious effect of sex hormones on the distribution of some parts of the fat layer in a typically female or male pattern, we have no idea.

Can I avoid looking puny after weight loss?

This might sound an odd question, given the aspiration to being thin and fit in our modern culture. But it is, interestingly, one often posed by people in positions of power. It has a greater importance in some cultures than in others. Views may be changing in the UK, where in times gone by, most company directors, most civic mayors, and most leaders would be large, imposing people. Elsewhere in the world, the phrase *avoir du poids*—i.e., to have gravitas, or power—could be applied to many of the top people. The best way to avoid looking less impressive despite weight loss is to undertake weight training to build up the neck and shoulders. And to have self-confidence. You don't need extra weight to give the impression of clout.

Quick Read

- Recognize the problem: if you have type 2 diabetes you have become too heavy for your body
- Write down your target weight: usually a weight loss of 33 pounds
- Recognize that food intake has to be decreased for 2–3 months: think when it may suit you to do this
- Discuss with family and friends: support is one of the secrets of success
- Decide: do you really want to do this?
- Prepare for action: clear the cupboards
- Action: do it

8

Enjoying Life and Staying Away from Diabetes

Golden Principles:

1. Only eat at mealtimes. Never between meals.
2. Eat purposefully. If food is eaten while reading, working, or watching television, far more slips down. Nor is it particularly enjoyed.
3. Commercial ready meals tend to be relatively unsatisfying and often contain added sugar. Avoid. There are plenty of easy meals made with fresh ingredients that can be microwaved in minutes.
4. Avoid sweetened drinks of all kinds.
5. Party, but pay back. Enjoy that special occasion. Life is for living. But after that, the next week is crucial: you must severely cut back.

The simple bottom line is: avoid weight regain.

Having worked so hard to get your weight down, you will be feeling better than you have for years, ready to embrace life with renewed vigor and confidence. And so you should. But do not relax too much! The period after rapid weight loss, when you start the switch back to more normal eating, can be a dangerous one. You will need all your resolve to keep to your goals and stay well. Stick reminders on the fridge and enlist friends and family to spur you on.

Remember, you will not be able to return to eating the amount you used to regard as normal. Keeping down your calorie intake is crucial, as is regular physical activity. However, you must bear in mind that the balance between food energy taken in and energy burned by physical activity is very delicate: a couple of extra mouthfuls of food can easily cancel out the effects of half an hour of exercise.

The rest of this chapter considers some strategies to help you plan your own approach and avoid the bear-traps that would cause weight regain and ill health.

What Really Happens After Weight Loss?

In Chapter 2, I made the observation that big animals need more calories than small animals. If you have lost weight, you have a smaller body to keep alive, and so you need less food. This is sometimes dressed up in scientific language—your metabolic rate has decreased. But that creates an aura of mystique; the real problem is the very human one of habit. Most of our lives run on autopilot—it would be exhausting to make new decisions every minute of the day—so we easily slip back into those deeply plowed furrows. Think about your food behavior: when do you find yourself eating? And with whom? How much do you usually put on your plate? How often do you cook using fresh ingredients instead of buying ready-made meals? It is vital to make yourself aware of your eating habits if you are going to make effective, targeted changes.

First, let's look at the experience of other individuals who have won through and escaped from diabetes. It is true that in any such group, the average weight will tend to creep up over time. But as is so often the case, the average does not reflect what is really going on. Behind the apparently steadily increasing weight we can identify several patterns.

The commonest pattern is to have a reasonably steady weight—one that has involved a clear change in eating habits and requires ongoing effort, and where everything seems to be okay . . . until a life event happens. It might be illness in the family or trouble at work, or any number of other things. Life does not run smoothly all the time. Naturally, the event fills the mind and has to be coped with. It is a daily preoccupation until resolved. And, in the meantime, all that focus on one's change of habits tends to fade into the background. Yes, it remains important, but it is displaced by whatever is immediately threatening the smooth running of life. As a result, weight increases quite rapidly.

Of course, in real life these sorts of events happen to different people at different times—although this is not reflected in the statistics, where everyone's weight is merely averaged over time. So the weight graph appears to rise steadily. There is an important message to be taken from this: you need to be prepared for how you are going to manage when life deals a hard blow. Being aware that stress can pose a problem is a good start, but you should have a rescue plan at the ready. It is too late to think about ordering a life belt when you are already in the water. This is one of the very clear lessons we learned from DiRECT. Rescue plans were lined up in advance. If someone gained more than 9 pounds in weight, we offered a liquid formula diet to help them get rid of the extra weight as soon as possible. Low-calorie shakes are a simple, effective option, but there are other effective ways of cutting back drastically on your calorie intake.

In our studies, about one in two people required at least one return to the low-calorie liquid diet, and some people required two or three. Tellingly, the overall weight loss at two years was very similar in those who had cruised along at a steady weight and those who had run into life events and needed an occasional life belt. Without recognition that life events occur, and that the stress of these makes us likely to regain weight, many of us would find our weight rising unchecked over the years.

A second pattern of weight regain is, as you might expect, a steadier increase—week on week, month on month, which means that something in excess of calorie requirements is being consumed. Sorting this out requires a clear-headed evaluation of what is happening. Sometimes an ongoing problem, such as stress at work, is chronically diverting effort from weight maintenance, and it may be useful to recognize this. Sometimes it is to do with food habits: eating between meals, or getting lax about portion control. You may have reverted to your old habit of putting too much on the plate. By hook or by crook, these behaviors have to be tackled. Consumption of beer, wine, and spirits may have to be restricted to weekends or partially substituted by zero-calorie drinks. Tap water is delightfully inexpensive—but the problem is often in the social pressure of buying rounds.

Another pattern of weight regain could be called the cruise holiday. Being exposed to prepaid food in limitless quantities is a sure recipe for putting on weight. Sometimes the weight gain is prodigious in a short time. It is easy to understand how this happens. You have been away from your routine, in a glorious escapist bubble; but on your return home from vacation you must be under no illusion that type 2 diabetes is ready to spring its trap. The weight gain needs to be recognized and dealt with urgently. You must go back to serious, focused weight loss for a planned period of weeks.

Steroids cause weight gain. We are not talking about anabolic steroids, which occasionally hit the headlines as drugs misused by some athletes to enhance performance. We are talking about the steroids that are essential for life and made naturally in your body. Given in high doses, these steroid hormones can be used as powerful drugs for some serious illnesses. These drugs directly stimulate the appetite. There is no easy answer to this unwanted effect. Seek advice from your doctor or diabetes nurse on how to avoid foods that are calorie-dense and ask them to help you find alternatives, or try a low-calorie liquid formula, as these products tend to produce a feeling of fullness. Fortunately, few people require high doses of steroids for months on end, and so once the storm has passed, undertaking a definitive period of weight loss will get you back on track.

And then there are the people who do not have any great problem in avoiding weight regain. These are often the people who had never thought about their weight in the past. They had just eaten according to their family and social habits and, if they had put on weight over the years, this had been slow and incremental and not associated with emotional and psychological ups and downs. On waking up to the consequences, this lucky minority can simply eat less on a regular basis without apparent difficulty. Probably they will not be reading this chapter.

Eating Food, Not Diets

Eating is a social activity. Many people eat in the same way as their close family. So whatever pattern of eating you decide on, it has to fit in with whatever else is going on at the table.

There has been much research into whether changing the amount of carbohydrate, fat, or protein in the diet is helpful. There are plentiful opinions on this; enthusiasts for any particular type of high-this or low-that can easily be found. In one sense, they are all right—any given diet may suit some people very well. So is there a best approach?

The basics of nutrition remain as valid today as they were when first worked out over a century ago:

- The body needs energy, but not too much, and this can be provided by fat, carbohydrate, or protein.
- Protein and some fats are essential, but in modest quantities.
- We also need vitamins and minerals. If you eat a reasonable variety of foodstuffs, true vitamin deficiency is relatively unlikely. Likewise, in practice, the only common mineral deficiency is that of iron.
- The bowels do best when presented with sufficient roughage.

The basics are genuinely simple. But we all differ to a degree regarding our genetic makeup and our learned behaviors. How often do you feel hungry, and what do you do about it? Are there some foods that you feel you could not do without?

No One Size Fits All

The common notion that there is one "healthy diet" deserves great scepticism. A single pattern of eating that is best for all individuals is improbable. Individuals differ markedly in food preferences and cultural habits. What is a heathy diet? Is it really the idealized plate of shiny vegetables often pictured in magazines?

Then bear in mind that your body sees little of the food you eat. It is broken down to its component parts in the gut, and these are then pounced upon by your liver. And as we know, it is your liver that ultimately decides how much of what kind of fat goes where, and what happens to the glucose. It gets first helping to decide which proteins to reassemble. But there is one respect in which what you eat does call the shots, and that is regarding the quantity. It is not correct to say that you are what you eat—you are *how much* you eat.

If your weight has gone up by more than a small amount since your mid-20s, then your diet has not been entirely healthy. Excess fat inside your body is a much greater risk to health than the kind of food you consume. Excess fat inside your organs is threatening, whereas the risk conferred by any given pattern of eating depends largely upon calorie balance. Almost all long-term studies of foods and health have been conducted in populations steadily gaining weight. That is a critically important factor overlooked by many offering opinions on how to eat for health.

There are a number of general approaches that might help you limit your overall calorie intake. Try these one by one. Only you can judge what works for you.

Low Carb?

Around 50% of the average British diet is made up of carbohydrate. Given that most countries in the rest of Europe eat 43–45% as carbohydrate, this may give pause for thought. After all, the UK is the Fat Man of Europe. This statistic is far from proof of cause and only an association, but the experience of many people suggests that moderately limiting carbohydrate intake may help with weight control.

Curiously, the hard evidence from research studies suggests that the effect of low-carb eating is relatively modest. There is a small benefit in the early months, in terms of both weight control and blood glucose control. But the very small number of longer-term studies to date show no benefit after one to two years. Why should this be? Probably because the basic premise that any one way of eating is best for everyone is flawed.

Most studies would assign half of all volunteers to low carb and the other half, say, to low fat. But in the low-carb group it is likely that only half of that group will do well. The other half will not like or will not be suited to low carb, and unsurprisingly will do less well. The same will happen in the group assigned to low fat—some will be suited to it and like it. They will do well, whereas others will not. Therefore, no clear benefit is seen in either diet. This is a fatal flaw in the design of these common, large studies. The approach is not helpful in discovering which pattern of eating may be most effective in keeping the weight off for you, or anyone else.

And then there is the issue of what exactly is meant by "low carb." How low is low?

Eye-catching short-term weight loss can be achieved by reducing carbohydrate intake drastically—to 20–50g per day. This means eating no bread, potato, pasta, rice, or other mainly carbohydrate-based foods. Certainly, some populations, such as the Inuits in northern Canada, have thrived on such a diet. Healthy life is undoubtedly compatible with a low-carbohydrate diet. After all, agriculture developed only around 10,000 years ago and during the previous 200,000 years of our evolution as a species, our ancestors simply did not have carbohydrate-rich foods.

For most people, low carb would mean eating 50–130g of carbs per day. That would allow you some starchy vegetables (a small potato, carrots, avocado), fruit, and perhaps a slice of bread each day. This has the advantage of being fairly achievable when eating with other people. You just eat very little or no potato or rice; and, when eating out, get used to putting most of the potato/rice/pasta to the side and leaving it untouched. That can be difficult for people who have been brought up to "clear your plate"—such an ingrained notion from the past.

It may suit some people to use carbohydrate restriction at a single meal. Perhaps no carbohydrate at your evening meal? Or just avoid bread or wraps at lunchtime?

Then, of course, you need to avoid ready meals, which often have sugar added. And as for fruit juices and smoothies—no, no, no! All contain concentrated carbohydrate as sugar, including the ones disingenuously labeled "no added sugar." Sugar is sugar, whether from fruit or factory.

Breakfast cereals are out. Why not go to work on an egg? The taboo on eating too many eggs is exposed as a myth in Chapter 9. And let's think about lunch. This meal doesn't have to rely on the ubiquitous sandwich or wrap—a slice of cheese, an apple, and some nuts are easy to carry.

Mediterranean?

The Mediterranean diet has received considerable attention. It is the way of eating most often found to be superior in comparative studies, provided it is moderately low carb too. This pattern of eating is based on vegetables, olive oil, and meats or cheeses. There are legions of recipe books on this topic. However, it does require more planning than just cutting back or missing out some foods. And the people you eat with regularly have to like it too. Otherwise, the problem of preparing "special foods" for yourself rears its more complicated head. Busy lives need simple refueling.

Intermittent Fasting?

Michael Mosley's very readable books have popularized the 5:2 diet—a regime that involves eating normally (but not excessively) on five days per week but minimally on the other two. Then, in order to keep weight steady following weight loss, he suggests you maintain a 6:1 approach, in which, for example, every Wednesday would be a fasting day with minimal food. Although some people do not find this easy to sustain, it is an approach that suits others—such as couples who follow it together—very well indeed.

One variation of intermittent fasting is to skip one meal every day. For those people who do not want to eat breakfast, and are comfortable not eating until lunchtime, this approach is ideal. There is no truth whatsoever in the catchphrase "breakfast is the most important meal of the day" (see Chapter 9). Others may prefer to omit lunch.

A further variation is timed fasting, where you eat all your day's calories within a specific time window. You could start with eating nothing before 12 noon, eat normally in the afternoon and early evening, and then nothing after 8 pm at night. That would give you a fasting window of 16 hours. But you could modify this to suit: eat nothing before 2 pm? Eat nothing after 6 pm? At present there is little scientific evidence to prove that intermittent fasting keeps weight down in the long term, but if it suits you and your family or friends, go for it. Your weighing scale will tell you if it is working.

Low Fat?

A low-fat diet to lose weight sounds superficially so obvious. Fats are the most calorie-dense foods. Certainly, avoiding excessive fat is a good idea in general. However, fat improves the palatability of some foods, and if you remove too much of it you can end up with a rather dry mouthful. The major studies comparing different diets have shown that the low-fat approach is as good as any other in keeping weight down (with the study problem described above). But beware commercial low-fat foods that have added sugar to make them taste better. They may be highly calorific and they will not satisfy your appetite for very long.

There is only one way to find out if a particular way of eating is good for you. Try it and see! You may really lock on to a low low-carb approach. Great. You may lock on to an intermittent-fasting approach. Great. Discover what really suits you for long-term health and happiness.

The key to success is finding a way of eating that you like and which keeps your weight steady. It must be sustainable for the long term.

A Word on Alcohol

Alcohol requires special consideration, because it is so calorific. One gram of alcohol contains almost as many calories as one gram of fat: seven calories in a gram of alcohol, to be precise, compared with nine calories in fat. However, I certainly wouldn't advocate a total ban on alcohol. For many people, it is a source of much enjoyment, and can be built into a way of life consistent with keeping weight steady.

Everything revolves around quantity. A home-poured glass of wine may contain 140 calories. That does not sound like much—about the same as a slice and a half of bread. But three glasses can just slip down, and they would bless you with 420 calories—a huge number if taken on a regular basis. Similarly, a pint of beer contains 200 calories. Downing five pints on an evening out adds 1,000 calories to your daily intake. No wonder a man's expanding waistline is sometimes referred to as a beer-belly.

The basic message on alcohol is to enjoy it in moderation—as long as you are honest with yourself about how much is going down and you can keep your consumption to within the weekly calorie envelope that will keep your weight steady.

Getting Around

The single, clearest finding of all the scientific studies on preventing weight regain is this: the best long-term outcome will be gained from a combination of avoiding excessive eating and drinking together with a sustained increase in daily physical activity. The benefits of regular, prolonged activity are discussed in Chapter 2. For people who enjoy exercise of any sort (dancing, aerobics, table tennis, running) that is wonderful—but only provided no extra food is taken because of exercise. Walk past those vending machines positioned for maximum temptation as you leave the gym.

How can you ensure a reasonable level of physical activity each day? Make it part of getting where you have to go. For instance, people living in London have the highest average step count of any city in the UK, because most cannot park anywhere near their place of work. There may be several reasons why people living in London also have the lowest average BMI in the UK, but one of them is that they do more walking.

But we can all build more walking into our lives. Absolutely anywhere is within walking distance—if you have the time. However, in practice, for longer distances, cycling can be good—anything other than sitting in a car or on a bus. People who cycle regularly have been shown to have longer, healthier lives, provided that the route to work is safe.

What Is in Your Cupboard?

There is frequent talk about our "obesogenic environment." It is assumed to refer to the pernicious combination of readily available, commercially produced high-calorie foods and our increasingly sedentary lifestyle. However, less attention has been paid to the obesogenic microenvironment of the home. Have a look at yours.

You may spend more waking hours in your home than anywhere else. If you are in employment, perhaps you spend 40 hours at work, but on most mornings, evenings, weekends, and some holidays you will be at home. If you are not working full time, you are likely to spend even more time at home. What happens if you feel hungry, or a little bored? Many people browse around to find something to put into their mouths.

Why do we do this? Over those 200,000 years of human evolution (and 3.6 million years of mammalian evolution before that), we have made searching out available food a top priority. In the distant past, frequent periods of food scarcity due to natural disaster or social upheaval made it imperative to make hay while the sun shone. Those who were best at this would survive the next cycle of crop failure or the lack of successful hunting. Critically, as we saw in Chapter 2, undernourished people are less fertile—just look at fertility symbols from any civilization and you will see the fat stores necessary for reproduction are prominent. For generations, being adequately nourished has been seen as a very good thing. Undernourished people tend not to pass on their genes. Continuing the species is an absolute necessity. Thanks, ancestors!

However, the fine specimens who seek out food most successfully have been rudely wrong-footed in the last 60 years. In this very brief period for *Homo sapiens*, food supply for much of the world has enabled even the poorest to obtain toxic quantities of things to eat. The full impact of this toxicity for the general population (unlike for the wealthy few) is still unfolding, and it is not good news. We are undergoing a gigantic experiment on the human condition. In our present environment, it seems the biological elites have become disadvantaged.

As a result of evolution, we have developed sophisticated mechanisms to promote eating behavior. Neural mechanisms in the brain and clever hormones acting on the brain encourage us to find food and eat to increase the chances of survival.

Yet we have evolved absolutely no mechanism to prevent over-accumulation of food energy. The problem is that we can still feel hungry, even though the body may be groaning under the influence of excess fat. Overall, if you are a person who has tended to increase in weight after the age of 21, you should be proud of your genes—but look to your environment and eating habits for salvation.

Let's take a look in your cupboards. Ideally there will be no biscuits. There will be no chips or similar snacks. There will be no cakes or sweets. Why would you voluntarily push calories into your mouth between meals? You know from reading the earlier chapters of this book that your body is designed to work just fine without any food for quite long periods. Between lunch and dinner is only a few hours.

How about your fridge? It is worth reiterating that the fridge should contain a jug of tap water (so that if you feel desperately peckish, you can drink a pint of cold, refreshing water). For special occasions or just for a change, there will be a few bottles of sparkling water. Your fridge will never contain fruit juice or fruit smoothies. These dangerous calorie bombs contain far too much sugar, which just slips down your throat and does not satisfy hunger. In our current environment, contrary to the claims of seductive advertisements, there is nothing healthy about fruit juice or smoothies.

Lucia, one of our psychology team, coined a nice term.

She worked on our Counterweight and DiRECT studies, looking at how our volunteers coped during the post-weight-loss period when they were getting back to normal eating. She found that, for most of them, this period was destabilizing and difficult. Buying more of some kinds of foods and avoiding others was a behavior challenge. Lucia identified the need to develop a new "foodrobe," drawing a comparison with the way we buy clothes and build up a wardrobe. This is worth keeping at the front of your mind. Sort your foodrobe. No easy snacks to tempt you; no sugary drinks; no commercial ready meals; just good, honest food to be prepared for mealtimes.

A Helping Hand

As John Donne observed so long ago, no man is an island. Nor is any woman. We live in a social network that is a whole subject in itself. The time that this really comes to the fore is when the world seems to be against you or when something bad has happened. Then support from your nearest, dearest, or closest is likely to be really important. When the going gets rough, such help of moral support is invaluable in dealing with problems that life throws up. Unpredictable events may upset how you thought your day was going to go. Then your best intentions may really be tested, and they may not hold up under severe stress. Picking up one's bruised ego and resetting those intentions is not easy.

Support from someone else is so helpful in these

circumstances. Psychologists call it "outside agency," and it can potently affect our behavior. Who can help? It could be your spouse, partner, friend, health care professional, muse, barber/hairdresser—the list of possibilities is endless.

In our very first study on reversing type 2 diabetes, I was surprised that I could not predict who would do outstandingly well and who would do less well. After being a doctor for four decades, reading people had been something I took for granted. It is useful to be able to anticipate a person's likely persistence in following advice. But this just did not work in our studies on diabetes remission. Then the penny dropped. It wasn't about the individual participants themselves. The research volunteers would often bring along someone to sit with them during the very long early studies, and I was able to talk with both.

An understanding soon dawned: the predictor of success lay to a considerable extent with someone's "significant other." Also, we observed a "buddy" effect. A volunteer's partner/relative/friend would confide surprisingly often that they too had lost weight. This was a clear sign that the cupboards no longer contained biscuits, chips, and snacks and that eating habits in the house had changed. Some enterprising individuals (outside the formal research studies) even set up self-help groups to capitalize upon the supportive effect.

We can't stop life stresses happening. But it is possible to ensure against such problems blowing us off course.

We Are Creatures of Our Environment

Why should obesity rates have soared in the last few decades? Often fingers are pointed and there is a great deal of muttering about sloth and greed. Clearly, any obesity genes cannot have become more prevalent in a generation or two. But everyone today is heavier than they would have been if living in 1980 (as discussed in Chapter 6). That usually includes the finger-pointers. The current environment promoting excessive accumulation of fat is a major problem for society as a whole. And the average weight of children and young people is likely to continue to rise if nothing is changed. Our research volunteers described, often very movingly, the trials and pains of living in our food-obsessed world: how difficult it was to get away from advertising, "recipe" talk, or counters laden with muffins and cake. This topic is large and beyond the scope of this book, but some key points can be summarized.

How about increasing legislation to regulate harmful food provision? Whenever this is proposed, well-meaning voices—and some less well-meaning—are raised against it. The mantra of "individual responsibility" is often heard. We should all have the freedom to choose, the loud voices insist. Yet the dramatic fall in bereavements due to road deaths that followed the compulsory use of seat belts and wearing of motorcycle helmets has not drawn comment from the same voices. Likewise, after smoking was outlawed in enclosed public spaces, major health improvements followed. These were far greater than any that could have been achieved by appealing to individuals.

So what about food? Surely if we can introduce legislation on the provision of toxic cigarettes, we could legislate against the provision of food in circumstances and calorie density that are toxic? The control of food is trickier, given that it is essential for life in moderation. Nevertheless, the motivation for a society to change its food environment should be potent. In the UK, the NHS spends an estimated £6.1 billion annually (2014–15 figures) on treating obesity, and type 2 diabetes accounts for the greater part of £10 billion spent on diabetes as a whole. But overall, the cost of obesity to the economy is far greater than this, considering lost days from work and other direct costs. It has been claimed that we spend more each year on the treatment of obesity and diabetes than we do on the police, fire service, and judicial system combined. Ouch. Taxpayers need to know, especially as rates of obesity look set to rise.

The effect of human obesity on the environment also deserves greater recognition. If a population of one billion people increased average BMI in step with the change in the UK between 1970 and 2010, it is estimated that the additional food production and transport costs for these heavier people would increase carbon dioxide emissions by 19%, or 1.4 gigatons per year. This is no trivial amount, as global carbon dioxide production is around 42 gigatons.

Societies face a big challenge. Major international food companies act to protect profits. They devote large sums of money to spreading misinformation and bending political ears just as the big tobacco companies did prior to legislation. Often this is done via impressive-sounding "institutes" or "research groups," introduced in the media as "the influential think tank . . ." Possibly one of the best-documented examples of a big company's machinations is the campaign run by a major manufacturer of sugary drinks to protect its sales in China, a substantial market. By establishing a research and advisory group and nesting it within a government agency via political connections, the company was able to subvert the public-health campaign against obesity. It did this by ensuring that the anti-obesity advertising campaign was restricted solely to promoting exercise with no whisper about food or high-calorie drinks. This health advice issued by the manufacturer carried the stamp of the government body. Sales were protected. The rates of obesity continued to climb. The full story, carefully documented by Dr. Trisha Greenhalgh, is a fascinating read (see Bibliography).

But is this wrong? In Western democracies, we expect companies to produce goods or services and make a profit for their shareholders. Clever marketing tactics are justified to achieve these aims. The problem lies not in commerce but in lack of regulation. Regulation would still leave a level playing field for competition. Clear calorie labeling of products, the limitation of fast-food outlets close to schools, a reduction in the calorie content of snack foods, and the constraint of mega-size or two-for-one bargains are just a few of the ways in which a new level playing field could be created for commercial interests to compete freely. At the present time, there are few politicians ready to face up to their responsibilities. Only a few years ago, a UK minister for health abolished the Food Standards Agency with its independent experts, substituting a body largely composed of representatives of the food industry. Since then, some of the resulting harm has been undone, but we can only wonder about what lay behind this decision.

The first step toward fixing our adverse environment will be to recognize the inappropriateness of political parties accepting funding from major food companies. The recent introduction of a sugar tax on soft drinks in the UK is a tiny step in the right direction.

5-a-Day for Legislators

Simple steps to decrease population level food intake. Several more are also feasible, but this would be a good start.

1. Restrictions on fast-food outlets operating close to schools
2. Regulation of added sugar and fat in processed/ready meals
3. Labeling of calorie content of single consumption items (e.g., fast food, ready meals, restaurant meals, individual cakes in coffee shops, cans of beer) that is clear, visible, and easy to understand
4. Regulation of supersize and bargain meals
5. Continuation of sugar tax on sugar-sweetened beverages

The Effect of Long-Term Success on Your Pancreas

The discovery that the pancreas was undersized in people with type 2 diabetes was a puzzle, as discussed earlier. Was the pancreas born small, or had smallness been thrust upon it by diabetes? We found a big clue to the answer in what was already widely known about the pancreas from another kind of diabetes—type 1 or childhood diabetes. Type 1 is caused by the genuine death of insulin-producing cells and an almost complete lack of insulin. It has been known for some time that the pancreas shrinks as type 1 diabetes develops. This was assumed to be caused by a lack of the regular big increases in insulin that have effects on growth (and maintenance of size) of all tissues.

Insulin is such a clever hormone that it not only controls how the body handles glucose, but at high concentrations also acts as a growth hormone. In normal health, at high levels after a meal, insulin effectively flicks a switch to maintain growth. Although usually we only think about the level of insulin in the blood, the levels within the pancreas tissue surrounding each islet must also be much, much higher. It is this huge level that may possibly help maintain the size of the pancreas. If the insulin spike were not to happen after every meal, we could understand why the organ might shrink.

Can the pancreas re-expand over a period of time if the surges in insulin levels are resumed? In our Counterbalance study, there was almost no change in the size of the pancreas over six months of follow-up. But in DiRECT, we have been able to analyze data up to 12 months at the time of writing, and found that the volume of the pancreas had increased modestly. So all is not lost if you have type 2 diabetes—and a small pancreas. Keep your weight down in the long term, and this vital organ is likely to increase in size.

Quick Read

- Once in remission, type 2 diabetes will stay away if you keep your weight steady
- The key is to find a way to live happily while eating only around three quarters of the amount you used to eat
- Build walking or another activity into everyday life
- Different people suit different patterns of eating—no one size fits all
- Moderate carbohydrate limitation may be simplest for some people; others are better suited to a Mediterranean (+ low-carb) pattern of eating, and/or omitting breakfast or intermittent fasting
- Recognizing alcohol as liquid fat is important in calorie control

- The obesity epidemic is environmental; it is not the result of a sudden onset of communal greed and sloth
- National regulation of food supply will be essential to make an impact on the epidemic

9

Don't Be Fooled

How do you know if something is true? Can you be certain that the information in this book is true?

Health stories are everywhere—in newspapers, magazines, on radio and television, online and on social media. Tips and advice about food and healthy eating are especially common. And they range from highly likely to be true to almost certainly nonsense. Don't assume that any one piece of information is correct; everything demands a questioning approach. Here are some ideas and ground rules that may help you to sort out solid information from misleading observations or baseless opinion.

Fallacy by Association

From the 1970s to the 1990s several large studies showed that post-menopausal women could decrease their risk of heart disease by 35–50% by taking hormone replacement therapy (HRT). HRT is clearly effective in relieving menopausal symptoms, but the decision whether or not to advise its use was heavily swayed by the likely benefit for the heart, especially in women with diabetes. By the 1990s. HRT agents were the most commonly prescribed class of drug in the United States. But all this was based on cross-sectional studies that looked at groups of women who were taking HRT and comparing outcomes with those who were not.

As discussed earlier, the only way to be certain that a treatment produces the benefits intended is to carry out an intervention study. In 1998, the first randomized trial of HRT on preventing heart disease was reported. There was no benefit—and alarmingly, a slight suggestion of a higher risk of heart disease in HRT users. These findings have been confirmed. So why did the original large studies mislead on such a grand scale? There are likely to have been several reasons. One is that women who sought out HRT tended to be healthier, wealthier, and behaved in other ways that decreased risk of heart disease. But the important point is that large studies that count events in different groups are bedeviled with unrecognized associations that may lead to a false conclusion.

Another classic example was the notion that eating a high-fiber diet had a major effect on protection against bowel cancer. This idea also arose in the 1970s, following observation of the notably high-fiber intake in African people living a traditional lifestyle and their very low rates of bowel cancer. The belief in a major causative link between low-fiber diets and increased risk of bowel cancer ran for quite a long time and still pops up from time to time. However, the lack of bowel cancer in those early observations in Africa was largely a result of few people surviving into older age when the incidence of bowel cancer rises sharply. Certainly it is a good thing to eat fiber-containing foods such as vegetables to keep the bowels happy, but this should be separated from the associated myths.

When reading a newspaper or watching TV—it does tend to be the media that broadcast these false cause-and-effect stories, rather than the scientists doing the collecting of data—look out for fallacy by association (appropriately shortened to fyb, as in "it's a fib"). How can one be spotted? There are several clues. Firstly, beware of very large studies. If a study has involved hundreds or thousands of people it may be merely a "counting heads" type of study. These can be very important in identifying patterns of disease, but are simply not able to prove that a disease is caused by some factor. Reasonable proof can only come from testing an idea. If you want to find out whether eating a certain food makes it more likely that a disease will develop, a change has to be made in a group of people and the effect of this measured. In other words, an intervention study is needed. To prevent other casual associations confusing the results, it is necessary to divide the willing volunteers into two groups at random, resulting in groups as similar as possible in all respects before they are treated differently. Then one group is given the food under test and the other, a control group, is asked not to eat it. Rates of developing the disease of interest are then measured in both groups. These real research studies are difficult to do, require a lot of money, and take a long time. But only they can give a clear answer to the question being asked.

One complete example of this is provided by the work of my colleague Professor Michael Roden, who is director of the German Diabetes Research Centre in Dusseldorf. He organized a large population study that found that people who ate a lot of red meat were more insulin-resistant than those who did not. The same study showed that drinking a lot of caffeine and not eating enough food containing fiber were also associated with insulin resistance. Almost always, epidemiological studies stop there, and the beliefs develop. Headlines follow and the lifestyle pages of newspapers and magazines spread the word. So does insulin resistance really increase if people eat a lot of red meat, drink a lot of coffee, and have foods low in fiber?

Michael is an all-round scientist, so he went on to do the definitive study. This involved dividing new volunteers into two groups at random, to ensure that they were similar. One group was assigned to eat lots of red meat, drink lots of coffee, and avoid foods containing fiber. The other group was instructed to do the opposite. Importantly, urine tests were carried out on everyone to check whether they were following the research guidance. It was very carefully conducted. And the answer? Eating lots of red meat, drinking lots of caffeine, and avoiding fiber had no effect at all in causing insulin resistance. Had it not been for careful scientific work continued over a long time, the myths surrounding red meat, caffeine, and fiber would have been perpetuated.

There was another important observation in this study that would have confused the results if there had not been a control group to allow comparison. Not only was there no difference between the groups but *both* groups became less insulin-resistant. This was because both groups had actually lost around 11 pounds in weight—without being asked to do so. This is a recognized phenomenon, called "the Hawthorne effect." When people take part in a study, even over a long period of time, they behave slightly differently. The message is that merely taking part in any study will improve your health whatever the treatment group you are assigned to!

The Hawthorne effect was first described in experiments done for very different reasons. Back in the 1920s at the Hawthorne lightbulb factory in Chicago, the idea was tested that brighter lighting increased productivity. It was discussed with all the workers and at first the answer seemed to be very clear: turn up the lighting and productivity goes up. But then a clear-thinking engineer went on to ask the workers to take part in a further study in which two randomly chosen groups worked under different lighting conditions. One group carried on with the usual lighting. The other had lighting that progressively decreased in intensity. And productivity went up in both! The fact of the matter is that people change their behavior when they know they are being monitored. This remarkable story does not end there. The workers were then told that steadily brighter lighting was being tested, and the lightbulbs were changed in full view every day. Everyone thought that the lights were very gradually getting brighter. But in fact this was a bluff: the bulbs were all the same. Once again productivity rose . . .

One of the investigators at the Hawthorne works,

F. J. Roethlisberger, wrote: "The consumer of knowledge can never know what a dicky thing knowledge is until he has tried to produce it."

Hang on, you might be thinking, Counterpoint did not have a control group of people with type 2 diabetes who, rather than going on the weight loss program, simply continued usual treatment. Why was the lesson of the Hawthorne effect not put into practice? The reason is that the size of the effect predicted was large—far greater than any change that might result from merely joining a study. If the Twin Cycle Hypothesis was to be proven, a fall in blood glucose all the way to normal had to occur, together with clear changes in the fat content of the liver and pancreas. Small changes in blood glucose or fat levels, even though statistically significant, would have disproved the Twin Cycle Hypothesis. In contrast, for studies that aim to test a new treatment, such as DiRECT, it is vital to have a control group, which we did. The people who had been assigned to the control group at random were identical to those assigned to the weight loss group in all respects—age, weight, male/female balance, severity of type 2 diabetes, etc. And in contrast to the gradual increase in weight that would have been expected in people with type 2 diabetes, the control group lost 2 pounds. Of course the effect size was so great in the test group that it eclipsed the small beneficial effect in the control group. The test group lost a lot of weight with many returning to absolute normality with a major difference between the groups. Hawthorne lives on!

How Large Studies May Mislead

Sadly, very large observational studies tend to attract a lot of attention. Even worse is the influence of what is inappropriately called "evidence-based medicine." While definite information is exactly what we must seek and use in medicine, the term evidence-based medicine describes a belief system that places a process known as "meta-analysis" at the top of the list of quality of evidence. Large, carefully designed studies can be important, and each deserves careful consideration. But meta-analysis is merely the process of adding together results from different studies—and believing the result of this must be correct. It takes little account of the vital details of the individual studies that a true expert would examine closely, such as the exact methods used in each study. It is also open to bias regarding which studies are selected for inclusion. Even worse, it ignores a vital practical point. The size of any one study is designed in a way that allows a clinically important effect to be detected, if present. An appropriate number of people are included so that such a clinical effect would be statistically significant. But by lumping together lots of studies that show no significant effect, meta-analysis allows tiny effects to become significant—in a statistical sense only. And such a minuscule effect may not be relevant to any one individual. While the headlines may shout that a certain food or drug can shorten life, in fact this could be by a few hours over a lifetime.

Observational studies on populations can provide invaluable information on patterns of disease. But knowledge about the cause of any outcome simply cannot be obtained at the same time. A specific intervention study is necessary.

Inappropriate interpretation of information becomes perpetuated by meta-analysis. Eventually, thankfully, this unfortunate belief system will drop out of common usage, but for the moment, the media and government agencies are bedazzled by large numbers.

Understanding Risk

Let's put risk into perspective. Many health stories in the news report that eating in a particular way or taking a particular drug will decrease the chance of developing some disease by a certain percentage. Let's say by 25%. That sounds persuasive and worthwhile, but in fact it is likely to be a small change. The reason is that the 25% figure is not about your real risk. It is the risk *relative* to some other group.

How does it work? Well, say your risk of having a heart attack in the next 10 years was 10%. People who start taking a statin drug have about a 25% reduction in risk. So the real risk to you would decrease by 25%. Your risk would actually drop from 10% to 7.5%. "So, doc, if I don't take the pills my risk is about 1 in 10, and if I do take the pills my risk is about 1 in 10?"

But if your risk of having a heart attack in the next 10 years was 50%, using a statin drug would cause the same 25% risk reduction—then your actual risk of 50% will drop below 40%. That is probably worthwhile. In betting terms, changing the odds from a 1 in 2 chance to about a 1 in 3 chance is pretty good. If 100 people with the same risk as you did not take a statin, then 50 would have a heart attack in 10 years. If a very similar group of people did take a statin, only 37 would have a heart attack.

So, what matters to you is absolute risk. If you can change it to a worthwhile extent, then some action may be useful. If, for instance, a new treatment halved the chance of getting a disease, most people might want to take the tablets. The 50% risk person is now down to 25%. But the 1% person is now down to 0.5%. Beware statements about percentage change in risk. What matters is the actual risk to *you*.

Effect Size and the Small Study

At the opposite end of the scale are the very small studies. However, they are potentially very significant, and make a huge difference to individual people. When Leonard Thompson received the first injection of insulin in 1921 and his type 1 diabetes improved, the world changed. Type 1 diabetes was uniformly fatal at that time but Leonard survived. The same happened when the first dose of penicillin was given to a child with meningococcal meningitis—a uniformly fatal disease was actually cured. The bigger the effect of a treatment, the smaller any study needs to be to prove a "significant" difference.

Of course there is always the chance that a freak

occurrence explains a dramatic response in one person, and confirmation of the effect on another person with a similar condition is required. However, the risk of these being a fyb is tiny. The main similarity between the first test on insulin and the first use of penicillin for meningitis is the size of effect produced—on previously uniformly fatal diseases. If a treatment genuinely has a big effect size, then only small numbers are needed to prove the point. And such a treatment is likely to make a big difference to every individual affected. On the other hand, if a drug study needs 5,000 people to show a statistically significant change, the benefit to any one person might be small.

When our Counterpoint study demonstrated normalization of blood glucose, liver fat, and insulin response of the beta cells, everyone in a group of 11 people had become free of diabetes. The size of the effect achieved was huge. Nevertheless, at the time, it was frequently dismissed by experts as being merely a "small" study. Did they have a point? No, but with one exception. Small groups carry the potential risk that they might not be representative of everyone with type 2 diabetes. However, we could show that the Counterpoint participants were entirely typical. And given that the intervention had a big effect that was both clinically important and statistically significant, the result indicated a potentially large benefit for most individuals. That cannot be said for most large studies.

Even though the practice of medicine is all about caring for individuals, at the moment big studies on populations are fashionable as a way to advance understanding. As a result, fybs are very common.

EFIs (Evidence-Free Ideas) and Bandwagons

Humans tend to want to believe—in all sorts of different areas. For instance, belief in astrology runs high, despite its improbability. Likewise folk cures, passed down by word of mouth, are often accepted without question. Wonderful claims for patent medicines have been made down the centuries, and sufferers from the relevant maladies have understandably wanted to believe in them. A recent study in the prestigious *New England Journal of Medicine* reported that people in the United States alone pay $13 billion annually for ineffective or fraudulent remedies.

As an example of this, the late John Diamond recounted in his remarkable book *Snake Oil* how friends and acquaintances would contact him with "certain" information of a cure for his terminal throat cancer. As an investigative journalist he was able to examine each claim. Sadly, none were true.

Once an idea gets out there, it is very difficult to dislodge, even if there is no objective information to support it. One first step in recognizing such a notion is to give it a name. As we are talking about an Evidence-Free Idea, let's call it an EFI (pronounced effie). Sometimes the EFI appears so self-evident that almost everyone accepts it. Sometimes it appeals to a group who then set about convincing everyone else of its efficacy. Occasionally one may be promoted for commercial reasons.

Some Recent EFIs

1. The Great Egg Demonization

When high blood cholesterol was recognized as being a risk factor for heart attacks, foods containing cholesterol were assumed to be bad for the heart. Eggs contain cholesterol. So the thinking went, we'd best limit our intake of them. Don't eat more than one per day! Better still, avoid all eggs! Pundits on healthy eating vigorously promoted the concept, which went unquestioned by public-health bodies. Even doctors with their feet firmly on the ground accepted it. After all, it seemed obvious. Cholesterol causes heart attacks and eggs contain cholesterol.

But wait a minute—let's ask some questions. "Does cholesterol cause heart attacks?" Certainly a higher level of blood cholesterol is *associated* with the risk of future heart attacks. How strong is that association in most people? Then you may ask: does eating eggs raise blood cholesterol? Again, there is no evidence of a causative link, although people who overeat generally also eat eggs and tend to have high blood cholesterol. The few people with specialist knowledge about cholesterol smile to themselves as the world rushes on. The panic about eggs is an example of an EFI.

Cholesterol is needed by all the cells of the body as a vital constituent of the membrane surrounding each and every one. We would fall apart without it. It is used to make bile salts, which help digestion. It is also used to make important hormones. Given this central role in life, it is not surprising that your body makes it for you. It is made in the liver. You can make up to a gram per day if needed. But if cholesterol is handed to your body ready made via food, then a sophisticated control system slows down the liver's production of it. Nature is always parsimonious, and the energy needed to manufacture cholesterol is conserved if possible.

A large egg contains less than one fifth of a gram of cholesterol (all in the yolk). If you eat more than five large eggs a day, there may theoretically be a problem—although it is likely that the body can deal with this by one of its myriad regulatory mechanisms. It also has to be said that unusual problems in controlling cholesterol can occur, so specific medical advice for individuals is important. However, there was never any satisfactory proof that eating eggs causes high blood cholesterol or heart attacks, or that restricting the egg intake of a population improves health.

The egg EFI persisted for decades, but at last has been officially debunked. The old slogan of the British Egg Marketing Board "Go to work on an egg" can be rehabilitated.

A postscript has to be added. Meta-analysis rears its ugly head. Yet another lumping-together of studies that merely report the age-old associations of egg eating has just been published (2019). The predictable headlines have appeared, even though there is no new information, just a recycling of old fybs.

2. Killer Fat

Another example of an EFI is the notion that a healthy diet has to be low in fat. It developed as a spin-off from an epidemiological study that counted up how much fat was habitually eaten and rates of deaths from heart disease. There seemed to be an association. This 1960s study was known as the Seven Countries Study. Indeed, it looked across seven countries, and found that heart disease was more common in the affluent ones. No surprise there. Then came the link by association: those affluent countries could afford for their populations to eat the fat of the land. But they also had many other differences in lifestyle. Even worse, it seems that information from other countries was not included. Had they been included, the association would have become much weaker. That became clear only some years later. Through the 1970s and onwards, successive studies found that low-fat eating itself seemed to have no effect upon life expectancy. But it was too late to affect the belief system.

Big problems occur when a scientific misconception is adopted by governments. The US government's first official advice on diet in 1977 recommended decreasing animal fat consumption so that it made up 30% rather than around 40% of the food eaten every day. It is likely that this advice was influenced to some degree by the heart attacks suffered by President Eisenhower. Yes! In the context of a country suffering what appeared to be an epidemic of heart attacks, clearly something had to be done. The association between the level of fat in the diet and deaths from heart attacks was sufficient to railroad a decision to name and shame the apparent culprit. Many lynch mobs have targeted the wrong man. But when governments get it wrong, the error tends to become the accepted norm—sometimes internationally.

Despite evidence accumulating against it for the past four decades, this particular EFI won't go away. Eating lots of fat certainly brings with it the possibility that too many calories will be consumed. However, as discussed in Chapter 8, some people find it easiest to avoid overeating on a higher-fat, lower-carbohydrate diet, whereas others may find limiting calorie intake easier on a lower-fat, higher-carb diet. It is the total amount of food that determines the risk of weight gain in the long term, and hence the risk to health. The human paradox raises its head again—biological facts do not necessarily determine human outcomes. All the personal and social influences on a person (habit, appetite, family and society norms, behavior of friends and workmates) play a part in determining what really happens.

Having debunked the notion that health flows from eating a low-fat diet, it has to be said that there are some subtleties in the debate about fat. Fat comes in several forms. The difference between saturated and unsaturated fat is explained in the box below.

What Is Saturated Fat?

As explained in Chapter 2, fat molecules contain long strings of carbon atoms. To make the string, a carbon atom has to "hold hands" with the ones either side of it, using two hands. However, each carbon has a total of four hands, and if the two spare "hands" on every carbon are filled—or saturated—with hydrogen atoms—then the fat is said to be "saturated." But if some carbons hold on to neighbors using two hands each (a double link), then they cannot hold on to as many hydrogen atoms and the fat is said to be "unsaturated."

If just one link is unsaturated, then the fat is called "mono-unsaturated." If a few links are unsaturated it is called "poly-unsaturated." Confusingly, mono-unsaturated fats (olive oil contains lots of these) seem rather better for the heart than poly-unsaturated fats.

Saturated fat is typically of animal origin. Unsaturated fat is typically of plant origin, such as in cooking oils. That is the brief explanation. In practice most sources of fat are a mixture of saturated and unsaturated.

There is reasonable evidence that the type of fat one eats makes a modest but worthwhile difference to health, with saturated fat being less good for long-term health than unsaturated fat. Substituting olive oil for lard, or eating more fish and nuts and fewer lamb chops can achieve this modest benefit for your heart.

But the facts may surprise you. In beef fat, just under 50% is saturated fat and just over 50% is mono-unsaturated. Olive oil is around 10% saturated and around 75% mono-unsaturated. Almonds are about 8% saturated and 60% mono-unsaturated. Tucking into your steak may draw tut-tuts from foodies who do not know that the fat in and around the meat is 50% mono-unsaturated.

Should we just cut down on all types of fat?

In Chapter 3, the fate of glucose was described. Anything in excess of what your muscle and liver are able to store or burn has to be shunted into fat for medium- or longer-term storage. And there is the rub. Because the process for doing this produces 100% saturated fat. If taken in amounts greater than your body is able to immediately use, all the extra carbohydrate is turned into the riskiest kind of fat, however brown the rice or whole meal the bread.

The simplistic notion that eating fat is bad for the heart and that carbohydrate foods are safer does not take account of the potential risk of swapping a mix of healthy and less healthy fats for 100% bad fat—in other words, the fat manufactured by the body from the excess carbohydrates. This process happens much more readily in people who are insulin-resistant, as explained in Chapter 4.

However, as always, nature provides an escape clause of sorts. Your liver will process some of the 100% saturated fat that you produce from any extra carbohydrate, changing a proportion to unsaturated fat. This capability to de-saturate the body's own fat varies between individuals. No wonder dietary studies often give muddling results.

What you eat may not be what your body has to deal with in the medium and longer term. The healthy glow surrounding various doctrines regarding what to eat may not be as real as assumed.

We have delved into details of how your body works, and it may sound complicated. However, the practical advice that results is simple. The balance of carbohydrate and fat that you eat is far less important than the total quantity, as carbohydrate regarded as healthy can be turned into undesirable saturated fat by your own body. And if your weight is creeping up, the undesirable fat may hang around and cause mischief. On the other hand, if your weight is steady through adult life, you are likely to be doing a great job for your health, whatever the mix of foods.

Another word of warning: for foods with equivalent calories, if the percentage of fat is low then the percentage of carbohydrate is likely to be high. Legions of low-fat foods, promoted as being healthy, contain increased sugar or carbohydrate instead, and thus add to the burden of saturated fat in the body. Supermarket shelves are filled with low-fat products, and few people read the labels to find out just what the fat in these products has been replaced with. Usually it is carbohydrate in some form—and the wisdom of this is highly questionable.

Recognizing an EFI is important.

3. The Importance of Breakfast

A steady flow of research studies on the importance of breakfast is published each year, usually in less prominent scientific journals but trumpeted in the media. Most show that people who eat breakfast tend to be slimmer than those who skip it. Yet again, this is an association, not proof of cause and effect. And it is quite different from showing that if overweight people eat breakfast they will become slimmer. Let's take a close look at how studies may be set up and what they actually show.

Unsurprisingly, these studies are often funded by the breakfast cereal industry, and usually work a similar dodge. Breakfast could be defined as a meal taken before leaving the house in the morning. Those people with more chaotic lifestyles tend not to eat in the house, but opt for fast food (biscuits, doughnuts, chips, burgers) during the morning or even on the way to work. These fast foods or snacks are typically calorie-dense and they do not satisfy the appetite for long. They also tend to reinforce the habit of eating between sit-down mealtimes and we know that snacking is likely to be associated with increasing weight. So by limiting what counts as breakfast, an association between being heavier and omission of breakfast is created. The fyb kicks in. A statistical tendency is created for heavier people to take breakfast on the hoof rather than eat before leaving the house.

The slogan "breakfast is the most important meal of the day" is a purely commercial confection but has been transmuted into "healthy eating." The idea has become embedded that regular eating of breakfast is obligatory for everyone.

Some people would prefer just to have a cup of coffee on waking and not sit down and eat. Provided they do not snack during the morning as a result, well-designed studies show that they have a lower daily calorie intake by avoiding an unwanted breakfast-time meal. However, for people who can't function without breakfast, it is far better that they do indeed eat before leaving the house. A boiled egg, maybe!

Individuals are individuals, and the myth that eating breakfast is mandatory if you want to be slim needs to be consigned to history. The golden rule remains—don't eat between meals.

Some people find this out for themselves. A compelling description of a personal voyage of discovery is contained in Terence Keeley's book *Breakfast Is a Dangerous Meal.*

4. Healthy Gut Bacteria Improve the Metabolism

Well over a decade ago, it was suggested that the huge mass of bacteria in our large bowels might produce chemicals that could affect our metabolism. It was an interesting concept, and clearly capable of being tested. Everyone waited for clear-cut studies to demonstrate how great an effect the bugs had. The years ticked by. Even at the time of writing there is no evidence of a cause-and-effect relationship in people. Evidence of lack of effect is beginning to appear. But the belief lives on.

Unsurprisingly, changing the types of foods eaten can allow some types of bacteria to flourish. Drastically decreasing the quantity of food eaten can change the proportions of bacteria in the gut—and of course blood glucose control improves. But yet again this is merely an association with glucose control and not cause and effect, as weight loss profoundly changes the metabolism in many ways as well as allowing different bacteria to survive in the gut. When studies have been done to add allegedly "good" bacteria to the gut, no useful effect on glucose control has been seen.

There has been little discussion about the bacteria most likely to be able to have an influence on the body—those which live under the layer of mucus, right next to the cells of the gut lining. These bacteria do not get swept along in the bowel contents and are hardly present in feces. One example is *Helicobacter*, which causes stomach ulcers. But it's the bacteria that are mixed in the feces, distant from the body itself, that are the ones counted in most studies of "bugs in your gut." If our local friendly bugs in our stools have any effect on metabolism, it is likely to be small.

Could I be wrong in coming to this conclusion? That is what a professor of medicine has to ask themselves every day. Knowledge is rarely black and white. Concrete evidence showing that gut bacteria do affect metabolic health may be just around the corner—but at present it looks very unlikely.

5. 5-a-Day

This phrase has such a ring of sense about it. Of course eating more fruit and vegetables must improve health. It has been seen as a low-cost policy with which to improve the health of the nation. It has become one of the most widely accepted beliefs about healthy eating.

One morning, I was woken by the radio news. The announcement that a major study of 5-a-day had found no benefit did not surprise me nor hasten my wakening. But then an expert was interviewed, who immediately said it was the number that was wrong and people probably needed to eat 10 a day. Gradually surfacing, I was dimly aware that it was actually April 1st. So I assumed that this would turn out to be an April Fools' prank. It was not. Experts, who have worked hard to acquire their framework of knowledge, are often the slowest to see that a basic error has crept in. Beliefs are dearly held.

There is objective information about how the 5-a-day campaign has changed food intake. National food surveys document how much of each type of food is eaten in the UK each year. Since 5-a-day was popularized, there has been no increase in the national consumption of cabbage. What a surprise! Nor has there been any increase in the consumption of other fruit and vegetables. None at all. What there has been is an increase in fruit juice and smoothie consumption. "It counts as one of your 5-a-day." Advisory bodies have been woefully slow to exclude these calorie-dense soft drinks from the slogan.

The idea emerged as a fyb. Cross-sectional studies clearly showed low fruit and vegetable consumption to be linked to worse health outcomes. It seemed to be a no-brainer. Then a number of intervention studies were done to measure just how great the improvement in health was after changing to 5-a-day. Well-designed intervention studies (to my knowledge) have failed to show significant benefit. For instance, in one meta-analysis, only three out of 18 cross-sectional studies showed a meaningful relationship with heart or stroke disease, but slight associations overall led it to conclude that there was a clear benefit in the 5-a-day message. There is a fundamental flaw with the concept. It assumes that portions of fruit and vegetables have essential health-giving properties. Antioxidants and micronutrients are mentioned—without evidence of relevance. Although all experts on nutrition are likely to agree that eating fruit and vegetables contributes very usefully to a wise pattern of eating a wide range of foodstuffs, the 5-a-day slogan has not been shown to improve health.

It appears most likely that it is not consuming a certain amount of vegetables or fruit that is important, but rather eating veg or fruit instead of more calorific food. The health associations observed in the cross-sectional studies presumably were in people who ate relatively less calorie-dense food but relatively more vegetables. Merely adding vegetables or fruit is unlikely to add to health, as the eating of calorie-dense foods just continues. On the other hand, not eating a cake but instead having an apple could improve health in the majority. Instead of more potato, maybe more leeks?

This clarification of best-possible information should not be taken to suggest that vegetables are not an overall good for most people. Perhaps the slogan could usefully be rephrased as "5-insteads-a-day"?

6. Magic Foods

The notion of "superfoods" that have special benefits is widespread. Celebrities sometimes attribute their body shape, their glowing skin, and their energy to individual foods. Magazines and papers love the concept. Cue attractive pictures of marvelous items of food alongside famous people. It must be true—just look at the picture. How the idea arose and whether it has actually been tested are largely irrelevant.

Did you know that blueberries were a superfood? I read it in a newspaper. The touchingly human wish to believe in food with powers is very potent. But I'm afraid that, despite the hyperbole about vitamins and micronutrients, this is almost certainly another fyb. The most likely explanation is that in any survey, people eating blueberries would indeed be found to be more healthy than those who did not. Try to buy blueberries in the least-prosperous areas of town where, for a whole slew of reasons, folk are less healthy. There are none on sale. In the prosperous areas, people tend to behave in many ways that increase life expectancy. Also, there is a much greater variety of foodstuffs in their shops. The consumption of blueberries—along with broccoli, pomegranate seeds, etc.—is just one of a range of behaviors that decrease the risk of disease. Do enjoy these delights if you like them. But so far, feeding blueberries to the people in the poorer parts of town has not been shown to improve their health.

Long-standing wisdom about eating a range of foodstuffs is of course important. Superfoods are not.

So What Is a Healthy Diet?

Given the most pressing health problems of today's population, some very basic concepts should perhaps be rethought. Certainly, all that we have learned in the last 200 years about the minimum amounts of vitamins, minerals, and protein needed to avoid disease remains correct. And, for most people in relatively affluent societies, nutritional deficiencies are not a problem if a reasonable range of foodstuffs is eaten. Some foods are both calorie-dense and unsatisfying, and that must be factored in. There is no magic to any food, and no food is healthy in itself. The devil, as we have seen, is not primarily in the type of food but in the quantity.

If Samuel Johnson were able to comment, perhaps he would say, in his pithy style, that a healthy diet could be defined as that which keeps your body weight stable throughout adult life.

Quick Read

- The bigger a study, the more chance that it could give misleading results
- Look out for fybs—fallacies by associations
- Look out for EFIs—evidence-free ideas
- "Low fat is good for you," and "eggs cause heart attacks" are EFIs
- 5-a-day really should be 5-*insteads*-a-day
- Breakfast is optional
- Once an idea becomes widely believed, it is impervious to factual correction by careful research

Recipe Section

In planning the original diet for the Counterpoint study, I knew that life was not solely about metabolism. The gut has to be kept happy. On a liquid formula diet, constipation is very likely. For that reason we advised adding in some non-starchy vegetables to provide additional fiber—and this worked. Also, people miss simply chewing—texture and crunch are good! We provided some simple examples to follow, but were very pleased when our research volunteers came back to us with their own ideas.

This section gathers some of the recipes devised by the people who know: those who actually followed the 1,2,3 approach to losing weight. They include dishes not just for the very low-calorie stage at Step 1, but also for Steps 2 and 3, when you are slowly returning to a "normal" way of eating, adding foods containing protein and a little carbohydrate. You could turn these recipes into a shopping list for those ingredients you don't have, and stock your pantry, fridge, and freezer in preparation.

A word on vegetables: even if you don't particularly like them you may surprise yourself. Just try some of the ideas. Ideally, you would nibble on various raw vegetables daily before starting the low-calorie diet, as the more times your taste buds are exposed to new flavors, the more they come to like them. Have an open mind and try things you didn't like previously. The aim is to find enough of a range of vegetables that you can eat and enjoy in order to carry you through the low-calorie diet and beyond.

RECIPES FOR STEP 1

During this stage, you can have a vegetable dish along with your liquid replacement shakes to provide some crunch and fiber. Here are some suggestions to get you started. Amounts are provided in the recipes. Use a small plate (8"–10" diameter). You can, of course, also experiment with your own veg and herb/spice combinations. On the other hand, you could keep things very simple—a green salad every day.

What Are "Nonstarchy" Vegetables?

"Nonstarchy" is a useful way of distinguishing the vegetables that it's good to eat from the ones to avoid, but of course all vegetables have small amounts of carbohydrate.

Green Leafy Vegetables

Lettuce and other salad greens	Broccoli	Cabbage	Spinach
Bok choy	Kohlrabi	Kale	Collard greens, laci-nato kale

Other Vegetables

Fresh or canned tomatoes	Sugar snap peas	Carrots & squash	Cucumbers
Bell peppers	Mushrooms	Radishes	Bean sprouts
Peas	Scallions	Onions / shallots	Water chestnuts
Okra	Artichokes	Cauliflower	Asparagus
Green beans	Zucchini	Brussels sprouts	Leeks
Eggplant	Turnip/ rutabaga	Celery root	Fennel

And Avoid

Potatoes, sweet potato, parsnip, plantain, yuca, corn, and beet due to their higher starch content. All fruit, nuts, and seeds—as these are far too calorific.

Dressings, Fats, and Oils

A small amount of fat adds flavor and texture to vegetable recipes. As they are high in calories, be very careful with portion sizes during this stage. Not more than once per day, you could add:

1 tsp olive oil	1 tsp oil-based salad dressing	1 tsp mayonnaise or crème fraîche
1 tsp pesto	1 tsp butter	1 tsp coconut oil

Herbs, Spices, and Flavorings

Add extra flavor and interest to veg-only dishes using herbs, spices, and low-calorie sauces. Which will you try first?

Basil	Lemon/lime juice	Garlic	Curry powder
Chili powder	Cinnamon	Black pepper	Ginger
Coriander	Soy sauce	Balsamic vinegar	Malt vinegar
Chinese five-spice	Harissa paste	Rosemary	Turmeric
Oregano	Thyme	Cumin	Peri peri seasoning
Tarragon	Dried chiles	Sage	Parsley

Kevin's Smoky Sofrito

Kevin perfected his sofrito during one of our studies, adding paprika to a classic tomato sauce to give extra smoky depth. It can be used as a sauce for other veg recipes, or cold as a dip for raw veg sticks. Make a batch on the weekend and keep it in a jar in the fridge to use as required during the week.

Prep: 10 minutes; cook: 1 hour 15 minutes for a beautiful flavor—can be reduced if you're in a hurry; makes 4 servings as a main dish (e.g., sauce for a whole meal) or 6-8 if used as a base or side dish (e.g., ratatouille)

INGREDIENTS

1 tablespoon olive oil
2 large onions, finely sliced
3 garlic cloves, finely chopped (or 3 tsp garlic paste)
2 red Italian frying peppers, seeded and chopped into ¾-inch pieces
4 teaspoons smoked paprika
1 teaspoon hot (picante) paprika
Pinch of salt
2 cans diced tomatoes

WHAT TO DO

1. Heat the oil in a large skillet over low heat.
2. Add the onions and garlic and cook for 15 minutes.

3. Add the chopped red peppers to the pan and cook for another 5 minutes.
4. Add both paprikas and a pinch of salt, stirring well with a wooden spatula.
5. Turn up the heat to medium and add the canned tomatoes. Stir well.
6. When the sauce starts to bubble, turn the heat back down to low and simmer for 40 minutes.
7. Remove from the heat and allow to cool, then blend to a smooth paste with a hand blender or food processor.

The following recipes suggest a few ideas for using this versatile sauce during the very low-calorie diet stage.

Carol's Ratatouille

Carol loved this vegetable recipe with rich tomato sauce and chunky, juicy Mediterranean vegetables. If you have some premade sofrito you can use it as the base for the veg, replacing the canned tomatoes and other ingredients here.

Prep: 15 minutes; cook: 1 hour; makes 4 servings

INGREDIENTS

For the tomato sauce (can be replaced with Kevin's Smoky Sofrito, page 248):

1 can diced tomatoes

2 teaspoons apple cider vinegar (optional)
3 garlic cloves, grated or crushed
¼ teaspoon each of dried rosemary, oregano, thyme, and red pepper flakes
Salt and black pepper

For the chunky veg:
1 medium red onion, chopped into ¾-inch chunks
2 zucchini, ends removed and sliced into ⅓-inch discs, then cut in half (or quarters, if they're large zucchini)
1 eggplant, top and bottom removed, sliced into ⅓-inch slices then cut into chunks of a similar size to the zucchini
3 medium tomatoes, cut into eighths
Olive oil spray (or 1 teaspoon olive oil)
A few fresh basil leaves, torn into pieces

WHAT TO DO

1. Preheat the oven to 350°F.
2. Spray an ovenproof dish with oil.
3. Make the tomato sauce (or use the smoky sofrito sauce in its place): Mix the canned tomatoes, cider vinegar (if using), dried herbs, pepper flakes, and garlic together, season with salt and black pepper to taste, and pour them into the bottom of the dish.
4. Lay the sliced veg over the tomato mixture.
5. Spray with oil and scatter the basil leaves on top.
6. Cook in the oven for 1 hour.
7. Serve in a bowl and enjoy.

Keeps refrigerated for 2–3 days. Alternatively, divide into portions once cooled and freeze for a quick and easy microwave dish during the week.

Celeriac Bravas

A lower-starch root vegetable replaces the potatoes in the traditional Spanish tapas dish, keeping the carbohydrate and calorie content down. Serve with a simple tossed salad as one of your vegetable dishes once or twice a week.

Prep: 10 minutes; cook 40 minutes; makes 4 servings

INGREDIENTS

1 large celery root
Olive oil spray
Kevin's Smoky Sofrito Sauce (page 248)
Handful of fresh parsley, chopped
Mixed salad greens, for serving

WHAT TO DO

1. Preheat the oven to 390°F.
2. Using a large knife, slice the top and bottom off the celery root so you have a flat surface.
3. Stand it on a cutting board and use the knife to slice down around the edges, removing the skin and any "gnarly bits."
4. Chop it in half and then chop each half into ⅓–¾-inch cubes.

5. Spray a sheet pan with oil, add the celery root cubes, and then spray more oil over them so they are lightly coated.
6. Roast on the top rack of the oven for 40 minutes (turning halfway through to ensure even cooking) or until golden and crispy.
7. Take the pan out of the oven and transfer the celery root to a bowl to cool slightly.
8. While it's cooling, place a few spoonfuls of sofrito sauce in a glass bowl, cover with plastic wrap, and heat in the microwave for 2 minutes or until adequately heated, stirring halfway through.
9. Divide the celery root among 4 bowls and spoon the sauce over the top. Sprinkle with chopped fresh parsley.
10. Serve with a handful of salad greens.

Courgetti Arrabbiata

Replicate a classic recipe using spiralized zucchini in place of the pasta, and your pre-made sofrito as the spicy sauce—just add some Italian herbs and you're done! Spiralizers are now widely available online or in supermarkets and home stores.

As a simple alternative, just cook the zucchini and stir it into a teaspoon of pesto.

Prep: 5 minutes; cook: 5 minutes; 2 servings per large zucchini

INGREDIENTS

1 zucchini, ends chopped off
1 teaspoon extra-virgin olive oil
Kevin's Smoky Sofrito Sauce (page 248)
1 teaspoon dried oregano
Handful of fresh basil leaves, roughly chopped, plus more for garnish
½ teaspoon red pepper flakes
Black pepper

WHAT TO DO

1. Use the spiralizer to shred the zucchini.
2. Place the oil in a skillet over medium heat
3. Spoon 2 portions of sofrito into a microwaveable bowl and add the oregano, fresh basil, and pepper flakes. Heat over high heat for a couple of minutes, stirring partway through.
4. While the sauce is in the microwave, add the "courgetti" to the pan and stir-fry for about 5 minutes, until soft.
5. Stir the sauce into the "courgetti," scatter some basil leaves on top, and finish with a grinding of black pepper.

Cauliflower Rice

A portion of cauliflower "rice" is carb-free and can accompany other veg ingredients in a variety of dishes where rice would usually be used. Here's how to make the rice itself.

INGREDIENTS

1 large cauliflower, leaves removed
Squeeze of lemon juice
Salt and black pepper
Herbs or spices of your choice (optional)

WHAT TO DO

1. Cut the cauliflower into quarters and remove most of the tough core. Chop each quarter into 4 smaller chunks. Blitz a few pieces at a time in a food processor until it resembles rice or couscous grains. If you don't have a food processor you could use the coarse side of a grater instead.
2. Add the lemon juice and season with a little salt and pepper. Adding spices, such as cumin, chili powder, or coriander, or dried herbs, such as thyme or oregano, before cooking gives this neutral dish a more aromatic flavor.
3. It can now be cooked in a few minutes by either microwaving in a large bowl covered with plastic wrap for 3 minutes on high (4 minutes if frozen)—be careful of steam when removing plastic wrap!—or roasting in the oven, which gives a drier texture and nuttier flavor, but takes a few minutes longer. To do this, mix a teaspoon of olive oil into the cauli rice, spread it in a single layer on a sheet pan, and place it in the center of a preheated oven at 390°F for 12 minutes. Stir halfway through to ensure even cooking.
4. Divide your cooked cauli rice into 3½-ounce portions. These can be kept in the fridge for 3 days, or in the

freezer for 2 months and reheated in the microwave or oven from frozen.

The following 3 recipes are ideas for using the cauli rice in your daily vegetable meals.

Cauliflower Tabbouleh

Traditionally, tabbouleh is made using bulgur wheat, but replacing this with cauliflower makes a super-fresh all-veg version. It should be bright green with the flakes of white "rice" barely visible, so don't be sparing with the herbs!

Prep: 20 minutes; makes 4 servings

INGREDIENTS

2 (3½ ounces each) portions Cauliflower Rice (page 253), thawed if frozen
Juice of 1 lemon
Leaves from 2 long sprigs fresh mint
Large bunch of flat-leaf parsley leaves, tough stems removed (you should have about 10 times as much parsley as mint)
1 garlic clove, minced (or use garlic paste for ease)
8 scallions, finely sliced
2 large tomatoes, finely diced
1 tablespoon extra-virgin olive oil
Salt and black pepper
Little Gem lettuce, separated into leaves

WHAT TO DO

1. Toss the cauliflower rice with the lemon juice.
2. Put the mint, parsley, garlic, and scallions in a food processor or mini chopper and whizz for a few seconds to make a vivid green mixture (this can be done with a knife and cutting board instead).
3. Stir the herb mix to the cauliflower rice. Add the tomatoes and olive oil, season with salt and pepper, and then combine everything well with a large spoon.
4. Serve each portion of tabbouleh with a few lettuce leaves, to scoop it up.

Harissa-Stuffed Red Peppers

Use your cauliflower rice as a filling and give it a Middle Eastern twist with the addition of harissa paste, made from chiles and widely available in jars. Harissa varies a lot in spiciness, from mild to very hot, so experiment and adjust the amount you use to suit your taste buds.

This dish can be served hot straight from the oven or kept in the fridge once cooled and eaten cold for lunch.

Prep: 10 minutes; cook: 20–25 minutes in oven or less if using microwave; makes 2 servings

INGREDIENTS

2 medium-large red bell peppers
2 (3½ ounces each) portions Cauliflower Rice (page 253), thawed if frozen

1 tablespoon harissa paste (or according to taste)
2 scallions, finely sliced
Squeeze of lemon juice
Bunch of chopped flat-leaf parsley, for garnish

WHAT TO DO

1. Preheat the oven to 350°F.
2. Slice each bell pepper in half vertically. Remove the stems and seeds and discard them.
3. Place them on a microwaveable plate and cook on high for around 5 minutes or until softened.
4. Place the cauliflower rice in a bowl and mix in the harissa paste and scallions. Add a squeeze of lemon juice.
5. Stuff each pepper half with the cauli rice mixture.
6. Place on a baking sheet lined with parchment paper.
7. Bake in the center of the oven for 15–20 minutes.
8. Serve garnished with parsley.

It is possible to make the whole dish in the microwave. Once the peppers are stuffed, put the plate back in the microwave and cook on high for another 8–10 minutes. Oven cooking chars the edges nicely, adding flavor and texture, which you won't get from the microwave. Take your pick!

Simple Broiled Eggplant

Eggplant have a firmer, meatier texture when cooked whole rather than chopped up. Delicious when simply combined with garlic and olive oil, and surprisingly filling.

Prep: 2 minutes; cook: 10–15 minutes; makes 1 or more servings

INGREDIENTS

1 small eggplant per person
1 garlic clove, cut in half
Drizzle of olive oil
Salt and black pepper
Salad greens and lemon juice, for serving

WHAT TO DO

1. Preheat the broiler to medium.
2. Using a sharp knife, hold the eggplant by the stem and make 4 slits at even intervals, lengthwise, just deep enough to pierce the skin.
3. Place the eggplant under the broiler, turning it as the skin starts to char and darken, repeating until all sides are slightly charred, 10–15 minutes.
4. Remove from the broiler and allow to cool slightly before removing the skin. It should come off easily.
5. Slice the eggplant in half lengthwise and place on a plate.
6. Rub the surface of each eggplant half with the garlic and drizzle with some olive oil.

7. Season with salt and pepper. Serve with some salad greens and a squeeze of lemon juice.

Helen's Garlicky Greens with Mushrooms

Prep: 5 minutes; cook: 10 minutes; makes 2 servings

INGREDIENTS

9 ounces kale (or any other greens)
1 tablespoon olive oil
1 garlic clove, crushed
1 red onion, sliced
7 ounces mushrooms, sliced
1 teaspoon red pepper flakes

WHAT TO DO

1. Steam the kale in a pan with a little boiling water for about 5 minutes or until tender. For extra aromatic flavor, try adding the crushed seeds of 4 cardamom pods before steaming.
2. Tip the kale into a colander to drain.
3. Dry off the pan, add the oil and, and heat over medium heat.
4. Add the crushed garlic and sliced onion and sauté for 2 minutes.
5. Add the mushrooms and pepper flakes. Cook for another 8 minutes, stirring frequently, until golden brown.
6. Stir the kale into the mixture, and cook until it's heated through.

Janet's Zucchini with Scallions

Prep: 5 minutes; cook: 11 minutes; makes 2 servings

INGREDIENTS

2 medium zucchini
2 teaspoons olive oil
3 garlic cloves, crushed
6 scallions, finely chopped

WHAT TO DO

1. Slice the zucchini into ⅓-inch rounds.
2. Heat the olive oil in a skillet over medium heat.
3. Add the garlic and fry for 1 minute, stirring continuously to prevent it burning.
4. Add the sliced zucchini and cook for 5 minutes, stirring frequently.
5. Stir in the scallions and cook for another 5 minutes.

Mediterranean-Style Artichoke Salad

Prep: 15 minutes; makes 4 servings

INGREDIENTS

1 jar quartered artichoke hearts, drained
1 jar of roasted red pepper (or use raw red peppers if preferred), diced
1 cucumber, seeded and diced
2 garlic cloves, crushed

1 small red onion, finely chopped
1 tablespoon extra-virgin olive oil
1 tablespoon dried oregano
Juice of ½ lemon

WHAT TO DO

1. Put all the ingredients in a large bowl and mix them together.
2. Cover with plastic wrap and chill for 1 hour to allow the flavors to blend before serving. Keeps in the fridge for 2 days.

Squash and Coriander Salad

This flavorful dish is especially good as a cold lunch the day after cooking. Use plenty of coriander and lime juice for a really fresh taste.

Prep: 10 minutes; cook: 20 minutes; makes 4 servings

INGREDIENTS

1 small butternut squash, peeled and cut into ¾-inch chunks
1 tablespoon olive oil
1 red onion, diced
1 teaspoon cumin seeds
1 teaspoon ground coriander
Juice of 1 lime
Chopped cilantro, for serving

WHAT TO DO

1. Bring a medium pan of water to a boil and cook the squash for 10–15 minutes or until tender when prodded with a fork.
2. Drain in a colander and cool under cold running water. Set aside.
3. Heat the olive oil in a skillet.
4. Add the diced red onion and cumin seeds and cook for 2 minutes, stirring frequently.
5. Add the drained butternut squash, sprinkle with the ground coriander, and cook for another 3 minutes, stirring frequently.
6. Stir in the lime juice.
7. Allow to cool, and sprinkle with cilantro before serving.

Helen's No-Noodle Chow Mein

Helen's dish is a good alternative to a more calorific take-out chow mein dish. Chow mein literally means "stir-fried noodles," but in keeping with the veg-only approach, here bean sprouts take the place of noodles. Helen comments "It's the most yummiest thing. Very tasty!"

Prep: 5 minutes; cook: 5 minutes; makes 3 servings

INGREDIENTS

1 pound bean sprouts

1 teaspoon sesame oil

3 teaspoons dark soy sauce

1 tablespoon olive oil
1 teaspoon finely chopped fresh ginger
½ garlic clove, finely chopped
1 carrot, peeled into strips using a vegetable peeler
4 scallions, chopped
6 mushrooms, sliced
1 small can of sliced water chestnuts, drained
1 red chili (optional), seeded and chopped
Dash of Worcestershire sauce (optional)
1 head bok choy, sliced into strips

WHAT TO DO

1. Place the bean sprouts in a bowl, add the sesame oil and 1 teaspoon soy sauce, and mix well to coat them.
2. Heat the olive oil over high heat in a wok or heavy-bottomed skillet.
3. Add the ginger and garlic. Stir-fry quickly for about 1 minute.
4. Add the carrot strips, scallions, mushrooms, water chestnuts, and red chili (if using). Stir-fry for another minute.
5. Add a dash of water—enough to loosen the mixture—then stir in the remaining 2 teaspoons soy sauce and a dash of Worcestershire sauce, ensuring everything gets a good coating.
6. Tip the bean sprouts into the pan, followed by the bok choy.
7. Stir-fry for 2 minutes and serve.

Easy Vegetable Curry

You can use any spices you like to make your own curry, and try different veg (cauliflower and spinach work really well) for variety. This version uses curry powder to keep things easy.

Prep: 15 minutes; cook: 60 minutes; makes 4 servings

INGREDIENTS

1 tablespoon olive oil
1 large onion, thickly sliced
2 garlic cloves, crushed
2 tablespoons curry powder
2 large carrots, thickly sliced
14-ounce rutabaga, cut into ¾-inch chunks
1 can (14.5 ounces) diced tomatoes
1¾ cups hot vegetable stock
4 tablespoons chopped cilantro
Salt and black pepper

WHAT TO DO

1. Place the oil in a large skillet over medium heat.
2. Add the onion and garlic and cook gently, stirring frequently, until the onion softens, 5–8 minutes.
3. Stir in the curry powder and cook for another minute.
4. Add the rutabaga and carrots to the pan, followed by the tomatoes, the stock, and 3 tablespoons of the cilantro, and give it a good stir.

5. Bring the pan to a boil, turn the heat down, and put the lid on.
6. Simmer for 30 minutes, stirring occasionally.
7. Remove the lid and cook for another 20 minutes, or until the vegetables are soft and the liquid has reduced and thickened a little.
8. Season with salt and pepper and scatter over the remaining cilantro before serving.

SOUPS

Lynda's Curried Butternut Squash Soup

Lynda loves curries and she experimented with different vegetables before hitting on this delicious combination of butternut squash and spinach.

Prep: 5 minutes; cook: 25 minutes; makes 4 servings

INGREDIENTS

1 tablespoon coconut oil
2 shallots, finely diced
2 garlic cloves, minced (or use garlic paste)
1 small butternut squash, peeled and chopped
1 tablespoon curry powder
¼ teaspoon ground cinnamon
Salt and black pepper
1 quart vegetable stock (homemade or from bouillon cubes)

4 handfuls of fresh spinach leaves or 3 ounces frozen spinach

WHAT TO DO

1. Place a large saucepan over medium heat and add the oil.
2. Stir-fry the shallots and garlic for 2 minutes.
3. Add the squash, curry powder, cinnamon, salt, and pepper to taste and mix everything well together.
4. Put the lid on and cook for 4 minutes, stirring occasionally.
5. Add the vegetable stock and bring it to a boil.
6. Turn down the heat, cover, and simmer for 15 minutes or until the butternut squash is tender (check by inserting a fork).
7. Allow the soup to cool slightly, then blend with a hand blender or in batches in a food processor.
8. Return it to the pan and stir in the spinach. Cover and let it cook over a medium heat until wilted, if using fresh, or thawed and heated through if using frozen spinach.

Keeps in the fridge for 3–4 days, or portions can be frozen for up to a month and microwaved or reheated in a pan when required.

Watercress Soup

Increase your intake of leafy greens without even noticing! This version replaces the usual potato with white turnip to keep the carbohydrate content down.

Prep: 10 minutes; cook: 35 minutes; makes 4 servings

INGREDIENTS

1 tablespoon olive oil
1 small onion, diced
2 small white turnips, peeled and chopped
1 quart chicken or vegetable stock (homemade or from bouillon cubes)
6 ounces watercress
Splash of milk
1 teaspoon grated nutmeg
Salt and black pepper

WHAT TO DO

1. Heat the oil in a large saucepan over medium heat.
2. Fry the onion for about 5 minutes, stirring constantly until it begins to soften.
3. Add the chopped turnip, cover with a lid, and cook for another 5 minutes.
4. Pour in the stock and turn up the heat to bring it to a boil.
5. Reduce the heat to a simmer and cook for 20 minutes with the lid on until the turnip is soft.

6. Add the watercress, turn off the heat, and allow the soup to cool slightly.
7. Blend in batches, then return the soup to the pan and add a splash of milk, along with the nutmeg and some salt and pepper.

Zucchini and Coconut Soup with Cilantro

Prep: 5 minutes; cook: 15 minutes; makes 2 servings

INGREDIENTS

1 teaspoon coconut oil
1 level teaspoon cumin seeds
1 small onion, sliced into rings
10 ounces zucchini, sliced
10 peppercorns
2 cups boiling water
½ teaspoon ground cardamom
¼ teaspoon ground cumin
Pinch of salt
Small bunch of cilantro

WHAT TO DO

1. Place the coconut oil in a medium saucepan over medium heat.
2. Add the cumin seeds and fry for 1 minute.
3. Stir in the onion and sauté until it turns translucent.

4. Add the zucchini, followed by the peppercorns and water.
5. Bring to a boil, cover, and simmer for 10 minutes.
6. Turn off the heat. Add the cardamom, ground cumin, and salt to taste. Blend it in a food processor or with a hand blender to produce a creamy soup.
7. Garnish with cilantro before serving.

Blended soups may seem just a bit too much liquid when combined with the daily meal replacement drinks, so here are some recipes that add texture as well as being incredibly tasty.

Chunky Vegetable Soup

Prep: 10 minutes; cook: 30 minutes; makes 4 servings

INGREDIENTS

1 tablespoon extra-virgin olive oil
1 medium leek (3½ ounces), cut into ⅓-inch slices
3 large carrots, cut into ⅓-inch slices
1 quart chicken or vegetable stock (homemade or from bouillon cubes)
4 celery stalks, cut into ⅓-inch pieces
6 spring cabbage, curly kale, or lacinato kale leaves, sliced
1 bay leaf
Dried herbs, e.g., thyme or Italian seasoning
Salt and black pepper

WHAT TO DO

1. Heat the oil in a large pan.
2. Add the leek and carrots and sauté for 10 minutes or until they start to soften.
3. Pour in the stock.
4. Add the celery and sliced greens, along with the bay leaf and herbs. Season with a little salt and black pepper.
5. Bring it to a boil, then reduce the heat and let it simmer for 20 minutes, partially covered with a lid.
6. Add an extra grind of black pepper just before serving and enjoy the juicy chunks of vegetable. This dish is even tastier reheated the next day.

Thai-Style Bean Sprout and Bok Choy Soup

Prep: 10 minutes; cook: 4 minutes; makes 4 servings

INGREDIENTS

1 quart hot vegetable stock (homemade or from bouillon cubes)
1 stalk lemongrass, cut into thirds and bashed to release the flavor
⅓-inch fresh ginger, peeled and thinly sliced
1–2 red chilis, seeded and finely chopped
1 red bell pepper, seeded and finely sliced
7 ounces beans prouts

2 heads bok choy, roughly chopped (or 5 ounces curly kale)
2 scallions, sliced
1–2 tablespoons light soy sauce, to taste
Juice of 1 lime
Fresh cilantro, for garnish

WHAT TO DO

1. In a large saucepan, combine the stock, lemongrass, ginger, and chilis and bring to a boil.
2. Reduce the heat to a simmer and add the bell pepper, bean sprouts, and bok choy.
3. After about 3 minutes, add the scallions and soy sauce.
4. Just before serving, add a a squeeze of lime and a few fresh cilantro leaves to garnish.

Remaining servings can be kept in the fridge for 2–3 days, or frozen in freezer bags when cooled.

RECIPES FOR STEP 2

Once you are through the intensive low-calorie stage, you can start adding in protein foods (and a little more carbohydrate) to the veg recipes you now know and love. A satisfying meal appears in place of a shake! Protein is the most filling part of the diet, and higher protein intakes are linked with more successful weight maintenance after a liquid low-calorie diet.

BREAKFAST

Spicy Breakfast Eggs

This uses the sofrito recipe from Step 1. If you do not have ready-made sofrito, you'll need to make a quick version as explained below.

Prep: 5 minutes; cook: 25 minutes (10 minutes if using premade sofrito); makes 2 servings

INGREDIENTS

Kevin's Smoky Sofrito Sauce (page 248) or quick sofrito: 1 onion, 1 garlic clove, 1 red chili (all finely chopped), 1 can diced tomatoes
4 eggs
Salt and black pepper
Chopped cilantro

WHAT TO DO

1. Heat your sofrito in a heavy-bottomed skillet (make sure you have a lid that will cover it). If making a quick sofrito, fry the onion, garlic, and chili in olive oil for 10–15 minutes until soft and caramelized, then stir in the tomatoes, squashing them with your spoon to break them up. Bring the mixture to a boil, then reduce and cook over medium heat until thickened (about 5 minutes).
2. Use a spoon to make 4 wells in the mixture.

3. Swiftly crack 1 egg into each well, season with a little salt and pepper, and cover with the lid.
4. Poach the eggs in the sofrito for about 5 minutes (or until done to your liking).
5. Serve up 2 eggs and half the sauce per person, with some chopped cilantro sprinkled over.

Lesley's Oven Frittata

Lesley regularly makes this quick and easy dish for her husband, Ray, who has now been in remission for over four years. He recommends it as a great way to use up leftover vegetables from the night before.

Prep: 5 minutes; cook: 25–30 minutes; makes 4 breakfast or brunch servings, or 2 main servings

INGREDIENTS

1 tablespoon olive oil
1 small onion, sliced
Leftover cooked veg (any kind will work)
4 eggs
Splash of reduced-fat milk
Salt and black pepper
1 large tomato, sliced
Fresh or dried herbs of your choice, e.g., thyme or basil

WHAT TO DO

1. Preheat the oven to 390°F.
2. Place the olive oil in a skillet over medium heat.
3. Fry the onion for a few minutes until it begins to soften, then tip it into a baking dish (around 6 x 8-inch), using a fork to spread it evenly. This also helps oil the dish to prevent sticking.
4. Now add the vegetables to form a single layer in the bottom of the dish.
5. Beat the eggs with a fork in a glass bowl or measuring cup, add a splash of milk, and season with salt and pepper.
6. Pour the egg mixture over the vegetables—there should be enough to just cover them.
7. Arrange the sliced tomato on top and sprinkle the herbs over.
8. Bake in the center of the oven for 20–25 minutes or until golden brown.
9. Allow it to cool slightly, then run a sharp knife or spatula around the edges.
10. Place a cutting board over the dish, then turn it over and give it a few sharp taps to turn out the frittata.
11. When it has set firm, cut it into four pieces and serve it with a tasty mixed salad or wrap it in foil to take for lunch the next day.

FOR LUNCH

Feta and Broiled Eggplant

This uses the broiled eggplant from Step 1.

Prep: 5 minutes; cook: 10–15 minutes; makes 1 or more servings

Simple Broiled Eggplant (see page 258 for full recipe)

INGREDIENTS

3½ ounces feta cheese per person, cubed

WHAT TO DO

Broil the eggplant and simply scatter the feta on top, drizzle with some olive oil, and serve. Done!

Kath's Hearty Veggie Chili

Prep: 15 minutes; cook: 20 minutes; makes 4 servings

INGREDIENTS

1 red onion, finely chopped
1 tablespoon olive oil
1 orange bell pepper, seeded and sliced
1 zucchini, finely chopped
2 garlic cloves, finely chopped
1 can beans or kidney beans

1 can diced tomatoes
Pinch of chili powder
Pinch of salt and black pepper
Handful of cilantro leaves, roughly chopped

WHAT TO DO

1. In a saucepan, fry the onion in oil for 2 minutes.
2. Add the bell pepper, zucchini, and garlic and cook for another 5 minutes, stirring frequently.
3. Stir in the beans, tomatoes, chili powder, and the salt and black pepper, and simmer for 10-15 minutes.
4. Serve the chili on top of a small roast sweet potato with some crème fraîche and cilantro leaves.

Chicken Skewers with Tabbouleh

This uses the cauliflower tabbouleh from Step 1. Marinated chicken is added for protein, and bulgur wheat replaces the cauliflower rice in the tabbouleh. Serve this with a green salad with olive oil dressing (3 parts olive oil to 1 part lemon juice, salt and pepper, shaken in a jar to mix).

Prep: 15 minutes; cook: 30 minutes; makes 4 servings

INGREDIENTS

8 boneless chicken thighs, each cut into 3 pieces

For the marinade and chicken:
2 tablespoons whole-milk Greek yogurt

2 teaspoons harissa paste
Dash of lemon juice
Pinch of salt and black pepper

For the tabbouleh:
7 ounces bulgur wheat (1¾ ounces per person)
Cauliflower Tabbouleh (page 255)

For the tzatziki:
3 tablespoons whole-milk Greek yogurt
½ cucumber, halved lengthwise, seeded, and finely chopped
1 garlic clove, minced
Dash of lemon juice

WHAT TO DO

1. In a bowl, combine the yogurt, harissa, lemon juice, salt, pepper, and chicken and stir well to coat.
2. Cover the bowl and refrigerate for at least 30 minutes or overnight—longer will infuse more flavor and tenderize the chicken.
3. Meanwhile, cook the bulgur in a pan of boiling water (about 1⅔ cups). Bring back to a boil then cover and simmer for 15 minutes or until most of the water has been absorbed. Drain off any excess water and leave to stand for 10 minutes before fluffing up with a fork.
4. Substitute the bulgur wheat for the cauliflower rice in the tabbouleh recipe, and set aside. The tabbouleh could be prepared in advance and used straight from the fridge.

5. Make the tzatziki by combining all the ingredients in a bowl. Refrigerate until needed.
6. When you're ready to cook the chicken, soak wooden skewers in water for about 20 minutes. Preheat the broiler to medium. Thread the chicken strips onto the wooden skewers.
7. Place the skewers under the broiler and turn them every few minutes until the chicken is nicely cooked (about 15 minutes).
8. Then use a fork to remove the chicken from the skewers and serve it on a plate with the tabbouleh and tzatziki.

Hearty Soup

This uses the chunky vegetable soup from Step 1. We added lima beans for protein and to make the soup more filling, and barley is a slow-release starch.

Prep: 15 minutes; cook: 30 minutes; makes 4 servings

Chunky Vegetable Soup (se page 269 for full recipe)
INGREDIENTS
1 can lima beans, drained
Handul of pearl barley

WHAT TO DO
Prepare the soup as directed through Step 3. In Step 4, add the beans and barley along with the celery. Proceed as directed.

FOR DINNER

Chicken Curry with Indian Spiced Cabbage

This uses the vegetable curry from Step 1. We add lentils to the curry for protein and slow-release carbs, and cabbage and extra spices.

Prep: 15 minutes; cook: 60 minutes; makes 4 servings

Easy Vegetable Curry (see page 264 for full recipe)

INGREDIENTS

4 boneless chicken thighs, cut into chunks
½ cup red lentils
1 tablespoon olive oil
½ teaspoon cumin seeds
½ teaspoon mustard seeds
0–2 green chilis (optional depending on taste), finely sliced
½ teaspoon ground turmeric
½ teaspoon ground coriander
1 small green cabbage, sliced; other sliced greens can be substituted if preferred
Juice of ½ lemon

WHAT TO DO

1. Prepare the curry through Step 2. In Step 3, when adding the curry powder, stir in the chicken and cook until it is seared on all sides, stirring frequently.

2. Add the lentils in Step 4 when adding the stock. Finish cooling the curry as directed.
3. Meanwhile, heat the olive oil in a large nonstick skillet over medium heat and let the cumin and mustard seeds sizzle in it for 1 minute.
4. Add the chilis (if using) and turmeric and fry for another 1–2 minutes.
5. Add the cabbage along with a splash of water, stirring well to coat with the spices.
6. Cover and cook for 4–5 minutes, then add the lemon juice and ground coriander before serving with the curry.

As an alternative the curry can be served with cauliflower rice.

Oven-Baked Salmon with Stir-Fried Veg

Uses Step 1 recipe: Helen's No Noodle Chow Mein (page 262)

Prep: 10 minutes; cook: 20 minutes; makes 2 servings

INGREDIENTS:

2 wild-caught salmon fillets
Splash of dark soy sauce
1 red chili, seeded and sliced
⅓-inch fresh ginger, grated
1 garlic clove, crushed
Juice of 1 lime
1 nest whole-wheat noodles

WHAT TO DO

1. Preheat the the oven to 350°F.
2. Combine the soy sauce, chili , ginger, garlic, and lime juice in a bowl.
3. Make 2 large foil envelopes by tearing off lengths at least double the size of your fish fillets. Fold the foil in half and seal on 2 sides, leaving an opening on the third.
4. Season the fish fillets. Place in the foil envelopes. Add a few spoonfuls of the soy mix to each before sealing the final side.
5. Place on a sheet pan and cook in the oven for 15 minutes.
6. Meanwhile, cook the noodles according to the package directions.
7. Make the stir-fried veg (see chow mein, page 262) and add it to the drained noodles.
8. Remove the foil parcels from the oven. Carefully pierce the foil with a sharp knife. Be sure to stand back while the steam escapes.
9. Transfer the fish to 2 plates using a spatula or fish turner, and serve it up alongside the stir-fry.

RECIPES FOR STEP 3

What do people in remission eat after a low-calorie diet? Just about anything except too much food, especially foods that are packed with calories. There are many good books offering ideas for tasty, satisfying meals, but here are some favorite recipes from previous study participants.

Pesto-Crusted Cod with Roasted Mediterranean Vegetables

Prep: 15 minutes; cook: 45 minutes; makes 2 servings

INGREDIENTS

2 cod (or other white fish) fillets
Mixture of vegetables cut into large chunks—red onions, zucchini, bell peppers, and cherry tomatoes work well
1 tablespoon olive oil
Fresh or dried thyme
4 slices multigrain bread, crusts removed
2 tablespoons basil pesto
Juice of ½ lemon
Salt and black pepper

WHAT TO DO

1. Preheat the oven to 390°F.
2. Pat the fish fillets dry with paper towels and set aside.
3. Place the veg in a bowl with the olive oil and thyme and mix well.
4. Spread the veg out on a sheet pan and bake on the middle rack of the oven for 20–30 minutes.
5. Blitz the bread in a food processor to make bread crumbs, then add the pesto and lemon juice and pulse until everything is well combined.
6. Season each fish fillet with salt and pepper, then coat them with the pesto mixture.

7. Bake them in a greased broilerproof baking dish for 11 minutes.
8. Remove the dish from the oven and place under a medium broiler for about 4 minutes, until the crust is nicely browned. Serve the fish with the roasted veg on the side.

Helen's Fish Pie with Celery Root Topping

Prep: 30 minutes; cook: 40-45 minutes; serves 2

INGREDIENTS

1 small onion, chopped
1 tablespoon olive oil
2 frozen fish fillets (cod, haddock, pollock)
½ cup water
1 red bell pepper, seeded and chopped
1 zucchini, sliced
Bunch of fresh dill, chopped
1 small celery root, peeled and chopped into ¾-inch chunks
2 tablespoons cream cheese (or crème fraîche)
Worcestershire sauce
Pinch of grated nutmeg
Salt and black pepper
1 tablespoon grated Parmesan
Green beans, for serving

WHAT TO DO

1. Preheat the oven to 350°F.
2. Fry the onion in the olive oil until it turns translucent.
3. Place the fish in a covered casserole dish with the water and add the onion, bell pepper, zucchini, and dill on top.
4. Put the lid on and bake in the center of the oven for 25 minutes.
5. Meanwhile, cook the celery root in a pan of boiling water for 20 minutes.
6. Drain the celery root, return it to the pan, and add 1 tablespoon of cream cheese. Mash, adding some casserole water for additional moisture if required.
7. Drain most of the remaining water from the casserole dish. Add the remaining 1 tablespoon cream cheese, a splash of Worcestershire sauce, a pinch of grated nutmeg, and some salt and pepper.
8. Cut the fish to break it up a bit and stir well to combine all the flavors.
9. Spoon the mashed celery root onto the fish mixture and spread out with a fork.
10. Scatter the Parmesan on top.
11. Return the dish to the oven uncovered, and cook for another 15 minutes.
12. Meanwhile, cook the green beans.
13. Serve beans alongside a portion of the pie.

Eggplant and Ricotta Rolls with Tomato Sauce

Prep: 15 minutes; cook: 1 hour; makes 2 servings

INGREDIENTS

2 medium eggplant, cut into into ¼-inch slices lengthwise
2 tablespoons olive oil

For the filling:
16 ounces baby spinach, blanched and drained
9 ounces ricotta
1 buffalo mozzarella
Pinch of grated nutmeg
2 scallions, finely chopped

For the sauce:
1 tablespoon extra-virgin olive oil
16 ounces cherry tomatoes, halved
1 garlic clove, crushed
Salt and black pepper

WHAT TO DO

1. Preheat the oven to 425°F.
2. Brush both sides of the eggplant slices with oil, then lay them on a large baking sheet.
3. Bake for 15–20 minutes until tender, turning once. Remove the pan from the oven.

4. Turn down the oven temperature to 350°F.
5. To make the filling, mix the spinach, ricotta, mozzarella, nutmeg, and scallions together in a bowl.
6. Lay all of the eggplant slices on a clean surface. Place about 1 teaspoon of filling at the bottom edge of each one.
7. Roll up each eggplant slice, like a cigar, around the filling, then rest them seam-side down on a plate.
8. For the sauce, heat the olive oil in a pan and add the cherry tomatoes.
9. Simmer for 8–10 minutes or until the tomatoes begin to break down.
10. Remove from the heat and stir in the garlic. Season, to taste with salt and black pepper.
11. Spoon half of the sauce into the bottom of a baking dish.
12. Carefully place the eggplant rolls, seam-side down, on top, and spoon over the rest of the sauce.
13. Transfer to the oven and bake for 12–15 minutes, until the cheese filling begins to bubble. Spoon the rolls onto plates. Serve with a salad or some green veg.

Kath's Roasted Sausage with Apple

Prep: 10 minutes; cook: 20 minutes; makes 3 servings

Kath's favorite recipes use lots of vegetables from her garden and are easy, quick, one-pot dishes.

INGREDIENTS

1 sweet potato, peeled and cut into small chunks
2 apples, cored and sliced
1 red onion, cut into wedges
6 breakfast sausages
1 tablespoon olive oil
1 tablespoon honey
Sprigs of fresh thyme
Green beans, for serving

WHAT TO DO

1. Preheat the oven to 390°F.
2. Layer the sweet potato, onion, apples, and sausages in a roasting dish and drizzle with the oil. Bake in the center of the oven for 5 minutes.
3. Remove from the oven and stir in the honey and thyme.
4. Bake for another 15 minutes, then serve piping hot with steamed green beans.

Carol's Parmesan Chicken with Garlic Stir-Fried Broccoli and Mushrooms

Prep: 10 minutes; cook: 30 minutes; makes 4 servings

INGREDIENTS

For the chicken:
4 boneless, skinless chicken breasts
Scant ½ cup whole-milk Greek yogurt

2 tablespoons mayonnaise
50g grated Parmesan
1 tablespoon garlic powder
Salt and black pepper

For the veg:
1 tablespoon olive oil
1 small onion, finely sliced
2–3 garlic cloves, finely chopped
1 broccoli head, cut into small florets
1 pound mushrooms, sliced
2 tablespoons soy sauce

WHAT TO DO

1. Preheat the oven to 375°F.
2. Flatten the chicken breasts (lay them on some plastic wrap on a cutting board, fold the plastic loosely over the top, and bash them with a rolling pin).
3. Mix the yogurt, mayonnaise, Parmesan, and garlic powder in a bowl with some salt and peper, and dip the chicken in it.
4. Lay the chicken in a baking dish greased with a little oil and place in the oven for 25–30 minutes.
5. 10 minutes before the chicken is ready, add the oil to a wok or skillet and fry the onion and garlic gently for 2 minutes.
6. Add the broccoli and mushrooms to the pan and stir-fry for about 5 minutes, leaving the veg with some crunch.
7. Finally, add the soy sauce. Serve the stir-fry with the chicken.

Tara's Tacos

Prep: 15 minutes; cook: 35 minutes; makes 2 servings

Tara loves this simple one-pot dish that is great for dinner parties/kids/big groups. Make it as spicy—or as mild—as you like! And Little Gem lettuce leaves replace the corn tortillas.

INGREDIENTS

1 tablespoon olive oil
2 garlic cloves, crushed or finely chopped
1 medium onion, chopped lengthwise into large segments
1 teaspoon paprika
½ teaspoon chili powder
½ teaspoon ground cumin
2 boneless, skinless chicken breasts, cut into chunks, or 10 ounces ground beef
2 bell peppers, of different colors, seeded and chopped into large chunks
7 ounces mushrooms, cut into quarters
1–1¼ cups canned diced tomatoes
Salt and black pepper
4 Little Gem lettuce leaves, for serving
Squeeze of lime juice

WHAT TO DO

1. Place a medium skillet over low heat and add the oil.
2. Fry the garlic and onion for about 5 minutes, stirring frequently.
3. Add the spices and keep stirring for another 1–2 minutes.
4. Add the chicken or ground beef and continue to cook, stirring every minute or so until the meat is sealed (the chicken has turned from pink to white, or the beef from red to brown).
5. Add the chopped bell peppers and mushrooms and cook for another 2–3 minutes or until the peppers start to soften.
6 Tip in the diced tomatoes, season with salt and pepper, and let everything simmer for at least 20 minutes, or longer for a richer flavor.
7. Spoon some sauce into the center of each lettuce leaf (you could also top with a teaspoon of sour cream and/or guacamole).
8. Add a squeeze of lime juice.
9. Wrap and enjoy!

Note: The cooking time can be reduced to 15 minutes if you have premade Kevin's Smoky Sofrito Sauce (page 248) on hand.

Kevin's Carrot and Celery Root Curry

Prep: 15 minutes; cook: 1 hour; makes 4 servings

Don't be put off by the spice mixes in this tasty curry. You can buy methi spices in some large supermarkets; and the jeera and haldi you can mix up yourself at home.

INGREDIENTS

2 tablespoons olive oil
1 tablespoon jeera spices: mixture of cumin seeds, brown mustard seeds, fenugreek seeds, and nigella seeds
2 red onions, finely chopped
2 garlic cloves, finely chopped
1 pound celeriac, peeled and cut into cubes
3 medium carrots, cut into slices
¼ cup red lentils
2 teaspoons haldi spices: mixture of ground turmeric, ground coriander, crushed cumin seeds, ground fenugreek, and a little ground black cardamom
2 teaspoons ground Kashmiri chili
1 can diced tomatoes
7 ounces green beans, cut into small pieces
Juice of ½ lemon
2 teaspoons methi spices: fenugreek seeds, cinnamon, fennel seeds, green cardamom seeds, and cloves all ground together

WHAT TO DO

1. Heat the olive oil in a skillet and fry the jeera spices for about 1 minute over medium-high heat.
2. Reduce the heat to low, add the onion and garlic, and fry gently for 15 minutes.
3. Stir in the celery root, carrots, lentils, haldi spices, and chili, together with 1 teaspoon salt and mix everything together.
4. Add 2 cups water, bring to a boil, and simmer with the lid on for 20 minutes.
5. Mash all the ingredients together, then add the tomatoes. Cook for another 15 minutes.
6. Finally, add the green beans and lemon juice and cook over low heat for 5 minutes more.

Allan's Ginger Chicken

Allan says he likes "fairly simple stuff," such as this kebab made with chicken pieces marinated in ginger and soy sauce. The recipe easily scales to multiple servings.

Prep: 15 minutes; cook: 15 minutes; makes 1 serving

INGREDIENTS

1 boneless, skinless chicken breast, cut into chunks
1 tablespoon dark soy sauce
1 teaspoon ginger paste
1 onion, roughly chopped
1 red or green bell pepper, cut into chunks

You'll also need: 4 wooden skewers per person, soaked in water for 20+ minutes
1 whole wheat pita bread warmed and split at the top
Shredded iceberg lettuce and sliced cherry tomatoes, for serving

WHAT TO DO

1. Mix the chicken with the soy sauce and ginger paste in a bowl, cover with plastic wrap, and refrigerate until ready to cook. Meanwhile, soak 4 wooden skewers in water for at least 20 minutes.
2. Thread the chicken pieces onto the skewers, alternating with pieces of onion and pepper.
3. Place under a broiler, turning every few minutes until cooked (about 10 minutes).
4. Remove the pieces from the skewers with a fork. Serve in the pita bread with the shredded lettuce and the tomatoes.

Tony's Alternative Sunday Lunch

Prep: 15 minutes; cook: 40 minutes; makes 3 servings

Tony has a garden and loves preparing food from fresh ingredients. He says that this, along with the smell of it cooking, adds to the pleasure of eating the meal. If you, too, have a garden, growing your own burns calories!

INGREDIENTS

2 boneless, skinless chicken breasts, cut into cubes
1 carrot, cut into large chunks
1 beet, peeled and cut into chunks
6 Brussels sprouts
1 parsnip, cut into chunks
4 shallots, cut in half
2 celery stalks, cut into large chunks
½ small turnip, cut into chunks
2 sage leaves
Pepper

WHAT TO DO

1. Preheat the oven to 390°F.
2. Place the chicken in the center of a large roasting pan and arrange the vegetables around it—this will keep it moist.
3. Add the sage leaves and a sprinkling of pepper.
4. Place the pan in the center of the oven and cook for 40 minutes, giving it a stir halfway through.

Kieran's Chipotle Sausage Casserole

Prep: 15 minutes; cook: 55 minutes; makes 3 servings

INGREDIENTS

8 good-quality sausages (less than 4g carbohydrate per 100g on label)
1 tablespoon extra-virgin olive oil

1 medium onion, sliced
4 garlic cloves, finely chopped
2 teaspoons chipotle paste
1 teaspoon ground cumin
1 teaspoon ground coriander
1 can (14.5 ounces) diced tomatoes
1 can (15 ounces) lima beans
1 red bell pepper, cut into ⅓-inch chunks
3–4 ounces green beans, cut into ¾-inch pieces
1 tablespoon tomato paste
⅔ cup water
2 bay leaves
Salt and black pepper

WHAT TO DO

1. Place a skillet over a medium heat and brown the sausages in the olive oil. Remove from the heat and cut each sausage into 4 pieces and set aside.
2. Add the onion and garlic to the pan and fry gently until soft.
3. Stir in the chipotle paste and the spices, then return the sausage pieces to the pan.
4. Mix everything together for 3 minutes and continue to cook.
5. Add the tomatoes, lima beans, bell pepper, green beans, tomato paste, water, and bay leaves, then bring to a boil, cover, and simmer for 40 minutes.
6. Serve with a green salad or some leafy veg.

Appendix

What Are the Other Types of Diabetes?

A. Type 1 Diabetes

This typically occurs in children and younger people. The peak age of onset is around 13 years. It is unusual after the age of 40 years but can occasionally occur even in later life. The start of this disease is usually abrupt, with symptoms including a strong thirst and a need to pass urine many times each night. These problems come on usually over a period of weeks, and most people start losing weight.

Type 1 diabetes has absolutely nothing to do with being too heavy or eating too much sugar. It is caused by the body destroying the insulin-producing cells with an autoimmune attack. We still do not know what starts this process. Unless insulin injections are started without delay, the condition is fatal.

Sometimes, especially in adults, type 1 diabetes can develop more slowly, which can make diagnosis more difficult. This is known as "slow-onset" type 1 diabetes, and it is often mistaken for type 2 diabetes. Blood tests can sometimes be useful in showing that type 1 diabetes is more likely than type 2 diabetes, but they are not 100% accurate.

In countries with a modern health service, around 8% of all diabetes is type 1. The figure is lower in less developed countries, where many people die from type 1 diabetes before being diagnosed.

B. MODY

MODY or Maturity Onset Diabetes of Youth is due to an alteration in just one gene. This abnormal gene causes the process of insulin production to be faulty. There are a handful of specific genes that can cause this—these have nothing to do with type 2 diabetes. Neither is this type of diabetes anything to do with being too heavy. Typically, many relatives are affected, and diabetes never skips a generation—parents, brothers or sisters, grandparents, and even young children can be affected. Because there are several distinct types, and specific genetic tests are available for some of these, definite diagnosis is usually but not always possible.

Around 1% of all diabetes is MODY.

C. Gestational Diabetes

This comes on usually between the 6th and 7th month of pregnancy. It goes away after pregnancy, but affected women are at high risk of developing type 2 diabetes over the next few years or in later life. It should be seen as an early warning. While in itself gestational diabetes does not cause long-term problems, if body weight is allowed to stay too high, type 2 diabetes is likely to develop within a decade or so.

Gestational diabetes affects 5–15% of women during pregnancy, depending on which level of glucose is chosen to define it.

D. Pancreatic Diabetes

The pancreas is an organ behind the stomach that contains the insulin-producing cells. Any serious disease of the pancreas can damage these cells and cause diabetes. The commonest such disease is chronic pancreatitis, which results in destructive inflammation of the whole pancreas. Cystic fibrosis also causes diabetes in many adults with the condition.

In pancreatic diabetes, often the effects of the pancreatic disease itself—such as weight loss and looseness of the bowels—are more obvious than the diabetes. However, diagnosis of this cause of diabetes is not usually in doubt. It accounts for a tiny fraction of all diagnoses of diabetes.

In summary, type 2 diabetes is assumed to be the diagnosis when middle-aged or older people are found to have a raised blood glucose and when there are no obvious clues to any of the other conditions listed above. Doctors know that nothing is certain in medicine, and reassessing the diagnosis is sometimes necessary. As time goes by, strong clues pointing to alternative diagnoses may emerge.

Acknowledgments

Behind every research project is a story about people. The adventures in science and medicine that are described in this book involve many individuals to whom I am enormously grateful for their skills, knowledge, and dedication. None of this excitement and discovery would have been possible without the people who volunteered to give up a slice of their lives, repeatedly lying in our scanners and parting with armfuls of blood. Taking part in clinical research calls for a high degree of altruism, and this is highly appreciated. I hope that this book reveals to each participant the whole picture that they helped to create. Many outstanding scientists have worked so hard on the projects described, developing ways of testing the body never previously possible. Each project also required a doctor interested in gaining experience of clinical research, to enroll participants, to carry out the hands-on special tests, and to gather the data. These diabetes specialists of the future spend a few years in research as a way of enhancing clarity of thought in clinical diagnosis and interpretation of data. They are all now consultant physicians specializing in diabetes, so their patients can tell you whether it worked! Several senior colleagues have collaborated, permitted research at the interface between different areas of expertise.

As my early work depended on taking tissue samples of fat or muscle, not without discomfort, I was excited to hear that techniques using magnetic resonance (MR) rather than needles had been developed at Yale University. Professor Jerry Shulman welcomed me to his team for a one-year visit in 1990–91. Without the insights and ongoing collaboration with Jerry and also Professor Kitt Petersen, type 2 diabetes might still be regarded as an incurable, progressive disease.

Dr. Parag Singhal spent a whirlwind year with me, and identified the big diabetes problem of the liver making too much glucose.

His careful work with people, backed up by the mathematical brilliance of Professor Claudio Cobelli of Padova, Italy, laid the basis for the Twin Cycle Hypothesis. Some years later, Dr. Peter Carey came to work with me before the Newcastle Magnetic Resonance Centre had been built, and our research volunteers agreed to travel from Newcastle to Nottingham (150 miles), stay the night in a hotel, have MR scans all day, and then travel back to Newcastle. Everyone who might benefit from the results of our research owes a big debt of gratitude to those altruistic people and to Peter, whose charm, empathy, and determination made the project a success. Peter Morris, professor of MR physics in Nottingham, devoted time and effort to make successful these first UK studies of muscle glycogen. It also helped to demonstrate just how valuable it would be to have an MR center in Newcastle.

Dr. Ravikumar Balasubramanian made the vital connection between fat in the liver and too much glucose being made in the same organ. These early Newcastle studies using MR relied on time borrowed on the hospital MR scanners. The subsequent MR research in Newcastle has depended crucially on Andy Blamire, professor of MR physics, Dr. Peter Thelwall, and Dr. Kieren Hollingsworth. They have carried forward amazing innovations and turned Newcastle University into an internationally recognised center for magnetic resonance research. The thrills of the scientific chase have been all the better for the huge fun of collaborating with outstanding people.

Dr. Ee Lin Lim joined me to carry out all the special tests for the people participating in the very first study of reversing type 2 diabetes to normal. Ee Lin carried out the demanding research study with a smile—even though a major wrench was thrown into the works at the outset. The government of the day, rather keen on regulation, had just introduced the bureaucracy that continues to this day to strangle UK clinical research. It took nine months of paperwork and oversight by various new official bodies to obtain all the permissions to do the work. That left just over one year to carry out the planned two years of demanding research. She did it! Her energy, skill, and enthusiasm were inspirational.

Dr. Sarah Steven took the knowledge about reversing type 2 diabetes to new heights, and somehow found the time to do several other research projects at the same time. She exceled in all respects, but particularly striking was her achievement of absolutely stable body weight in her research participants for six months following the rapid weight loss. The sheer hard work and empathy, together with culinary knowledge, were exemplary. I also thank Lucia Rehackova, psychologist, who joined Sarah to find out what people thought about undergoing and maintaining weight loss. Dr. Mavin Macauley, while investigating other aspects of liver fat in diabetes, made the astounding discovery that the pancreas is small and irregular in type 2 diabetes. My surgical colleagues Mr. Peter Small and Mr. Sean Woodcock were enormously helpful in planning and executing our research on bariatric surgery.

Dr. Carl Peters from Auckland, New Zealand, made the bold jump to Newcastle to work on the Diabetes Remission Clinical Trial (DiRECT). As a four-times dinghy sailing champion of New Zealand, he knew a thing or two about skill, determination, and hard work. He initiated the detailed scientific studies and brilliantly carried the study forward. Dr. Sviatlana Zhyszneuskaya then took over. She worked so hard for three years to complete the vital clinical tests, as well as encouraging and supporting our noble research volunteers.

The scientific work on finding the cause of type 2 diabetes and exactly what happens to bring the body back to normal depended upon developing and carrying out difficult laboratory tests. Dr. Ahmad Al-Mrabeh took the work to new heights with his scientific ability and ingenuity. This was not always straightforward, as world events impinge upon science. Ahmad came from Syria to the UK to undertake PhD studies, completed these over several years—but was then marooned here by the outbreak of war back home. His fantastic scientific contribution to reversing type 2 diabetes was carried forward at the same time as six years of battling extradition by an automatic bureaucratic process. Fortunately for people with diabetes, for UK science and for Ahmad, the long struggle with the immigration process to contribute further to diabetes research has been won.

Professor Mike Lean of the University of Glasgow is one of the world's leading experts in obesity, nutrition, and diabetes and the Diabetes Remission Clinical Trial (DiRECT) is a triumph of our collaboration. It was essential to find out if the means of achieving remission of type 2 diabetes could be rolled out in routine NHS practice, and our combined expertise was needed to make the trial a success. The full story of DiRECT (a large team effort) is yet to be told, and this book is focused upon the early studies on the how and why of reversal of type 2 diabetes. I must make special mention of Alison Barnes, who joined DiRECT as senior research dietitian to train routine NHS staff in the Newcastle area. Her energy and professionalism in transferring skills to primary care nurses or dietitians were legendary. Alison has also contributed in many ways to spread knowledge of how to achieve remission of type 2 diabetes in the UK. She had the bright idea of including in this book recipe ideas collected from our research participants and the recipe section is largely her work.

I am very grateful to Professors Ashley Adamson, Falko Sniehotta, and John Mathers of the Institute of Health and Society, Newcastle University, for advice and support. My longstanding colleague, Professor Naveed Sattar of the University of Glasgow, has been a much-appreciated touchstone for discussion and honing of ideas over many years. Similarly, collaboration with Professor Rury Holman of Oxford University was extremely valuable in developing the Personal Fat Threshold concept.

In tackling big questions of medicine, it is essential to know your enemy. Most of my insights into diabetes were gained by talking with patients. This was hugely amplified by discussions with and insights from Deirdre Kyne-Grzebalski, diabetes specialist nurse colleague throughout most of my clinical career. Professor Sir George Alberti created the fabulously fertile diabetes research scene in Newcastle and was my research supervisor in the early 1980s, and I appreciate very much his enormous influence upon my work. I have benefitted from discussions with my consultant colleagues, especially Professor Sally Marshall, over the years.

The Diabetes UK Research Committee had the imagination and foresight to fund the Counterpoint study, which revealed the cause of type 2 diabetes and why it is a reversible condition.

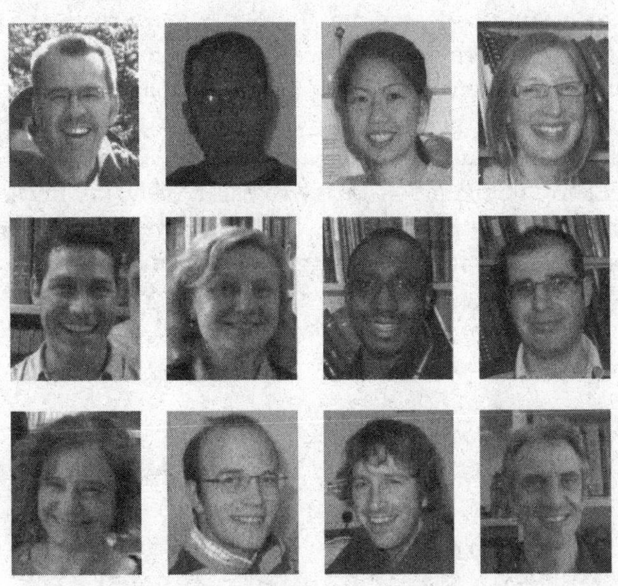

The main heroes of the research. From top left: Dr. Peter Carey, Dr. Ravi Balasubramanian, Dr. Ee Lin Lim, Dr. Sarah Steven, Dr. Carl Peters, Dr. Sviatlana Zhuzyneuskaya, Dr. Mavin Macaulay, Dr. Ahmad Al-Mrabeh, Miss Alison Barnes, Dr. Kieren Hollingsworth, Dr. Pete Thelwall and Professor Andy Blamire.

That was the essential step that opened up all the subsequent research and deserves widespread recognition. Diabetes UK also funded the DiRECT study, which tested general applicability of achieving remission in primary care. I have no commercial ties. I serve on a UK government working group (Scientific Advisory Committee on Nutrition, jointly with Diabetes UK), assessing the published evidence about low-carbohydrate diets. The views expressed in this book are personal and not those of the working group.

I am particularly grateful to two people for reading the manuscript, James Taylor (son, and consultant physician) and Paul Stein (friend since primary school and enthusiast for all things Viking). They suggested improvements and spotted obtuse comments and non-sequiturs. Those that remain are my fault entirely! Transforming ideas and information into a book has been greatly assisted by Jaime Marshall, publishing agent, and Aurea Carpenter, publisher.

The work would not have been possible without long hours of absence from family—usually absent in body, but frequently absent in mind. I am so grateful for the very long-standing forbearance and support of Aileen, my wife, and sons James, Donald, Alasdair, and Duncan.

Permissions

Permission to reproduce data and figures is gratefully acknowledged as follows:

Figure 2.5a - *American Journal of Physiology* (Taylor R et al, Direct measurement of change in muscle glycogen concentration after a mixed meal in normal subjects. 1993; 265: E224–229)

Figure 4.3 - *Lancet* (Tabak AG, et al. Trajectories of glycaemia, insulin sensitivity, and insulin secretion before diagnosis of type 2 diabetes: an analysis from the Whitehall II study. 2009; 373 (9682): 2215–21)

Figure 4.4 - *Diabetes* (Sattar N, et al. Serial metabolic measurements and conversion to type 2 diabetes in the west of Scotland coronary prevention study: specific elevations in alanine aminotransferase and triglycerides suggest hepatic fat accumulation as a potential contributing factor. 2007; 56(4): 984–91)

Figures 5.1 and 5.2—Diabetologia (Taylor R. Pathogenesis of Type 2 Diabetes: Tracing the reverse path from cure to cause. 2008; 51: 1781–1789)

Figures 5.3 and 5.5—Diabetologia (Lim EL, et al. Reversal of type 2 diabetes: Normalisation of beta cell function in association with decreased pancreas and liver triacylglycerol. 2011; 54: 2506–2514)

Figure 6.1 - Newcastle Public Library

Figure 6.2 - Annals of Human Biology (Rosenbaum S, et al, A survey of heights and weights of adults in Great Britain, 1985; 12, 115–127)

Figure 6.3 - Davies, S.C. "Annual Report of the Chief Medical Officer, Surveillance Volume, 2012: On the State of the Public's Health" London: Department of Health (2014)

Figure 6.4—*Quarterly Journal of Medicine* (Taylor R & Holman R, Normal Weight Individuals who Develop Type 2 Diabetes: The Personal Fat Threshold, 2015; 128: 405–410)

Quotations on pages 176–177 and 183 - Diabetic Medicine (Rehackova L, et al. Acceptability of a very-low-energy diet in Type 2 diabetes: patient experiences and behaviour regulation 2017; 34: 1554–1567)

Bibliography

The author's research is summarized with links to online lectures and publications at: https://go.ncl.ac.uk/diabetes-reversal

Chapter 2

Metabolic Regulation: A Human Perspective. Frayn, K.F. Wiley-Blackwell 3rd Ed 2012

Shadows on the Wasteland. Stroud, M. Overlook Press, 1996

Compendium of Physical Activities: Classification of energy costs of human physical activities. Ainsworth, B.E. et al. Medicine and Science in Sports and Exercise 1993, 25: 71–80

Chapter 3

Annual Report of the Chief Medical Officer 2012: Chapter 5—Diet, physical activity and obesity. https://assets.publishing.service.gov.uk/government/uploads/system/uploads/attachment_data/file/298297/cmo-report-2012.pdf

Regulation of endogenous glucose production after a mixed meal in Type 2 diabetes. Singhal, P, et al. *American Journal of Physiology* 2002; 283: E275–83. https://www.physiology.org/doi/pdf/10.1152/ajpendo.00424.2001

Direct measurement of change in muscle glycogen concentration after a mixed meal in normal subjects. Taylor, R, et al. *American Journal of Physiology* 1993; 265: E224–229 https://www.physiology.org/doi/pdf/10.1152/ajpendo.1993.265.2.E224

Direct assessment of liver glycogen storage and regulation of glucose homeostasis after a mixed meal in normal subjects. Taylor R, et al. *Journal of Clinical Investigation* 1996; 97:126–132. https://www.ncbi.nlm.nih.gov/pmc/articles/PMC507070/pdf/970126.pdf

Altered volume, morphology and composition of the pancreas in type 2 diabetes. Macauley, M, et al. PLOS One 2015 May 7;10(5):e0126825. https://journals.plos.org/plosone/article/file?id=10.1371/journal.pone.0126825&type=printable

Quantification of intrapancreatic fat in type 2 diabetes by MRI. Al-Mrabeh, A, et al. PLOS One 2017 Apr 3;12(4):e0174660. https://journals.plos.org/plosone/article/file?id=10.1371/journal.pone.0174660&type=printable

Direct assessment of muscle glycogen storage after mixed meals in normal and type 2 diabetic subjects. Carey, P.E., et al. *American Journal of Physiology* 2003; 284: E286–294. https://www.physiology.org/doi/pdf/10.1152/ajpendo.00471.2002

Chapter 4

Increased de novo lipogenesis is a distinct characteristic of individuals with nonalcoholic fatty liver disease. Lambert, J.E., et al. *Gastroenterology* 2014; 146: 726–35. https://www.ncbi.nlm.nih.gov/pmc/articles/PMC6276362/pdf/nihms-547033.pdf

Trajectories of glycaemia, insulin sensitivity, and insulin secretion before diagnosis of type 2 diabetes: an analysis from the Whitehall II study. Tabak, A.G., et al. *Lancet* 2009; 373: 2215–21. https://reader.elsevier.com/reader/sd/pii/S014067360960619X?token=7F49A5E4CCAFDD5FC3B2E50944F04F7CF400A402B86CDB2588E7868781090CA289B6E7C268BD5FFB0E1AB6F1EB409874

Serial metabolic measurements and conversion to type 2 diabetes in the west of Scotland coronary prevention study: specific elevations in alanine aminotransferase and triglycerides suggest hepatic fat accumulation as a potential contributing factor. Sattar, N., et al. *Diabetes* 2007; 56: 984–91. https://diabetes.diabetesjournals.org/content/diabetes/56/4/984.full.pdf

Chapter 5

Reversal of nonalcoholic hepatic steatosis, hepatic insulin resistance, and hyperglycemia by moderate weight reduction in patients with type 2 diabetes. Petersen, K.F., et al. *Diabetes* 2005; 54: 603–8. https://diabetes.diabetesjournals.org/content/diabetes/54/3/603.full.pdf

Pathogenesis of Type 2 Diabetes: Tracing the reverse path from cure to cause. Taylor R. *Diabetologia* 2008; 51: 1781–1789. https://link.springer.com/content/pdf/10.1007%2Fs00125-008-1116-7.pdf

Reversal of type 2 diabetes: Normalisation of beta cell function in association with decreased pancreas and liver triacylglycerol. Lim, E.L., et al. *Diabetologia* 2011; 54: 2506–2514. https://link.springer.com/content/pdf/10.1007%2Fs00125-011-2204-7.pdf

Population response to information on reversibility of type 2 diabetes. Steven, S., et al. *Diabetic Medicine* 2013; 30(4):e135-8. https://onlinelibrary.wiley.com/doi/epdf/10.1111/dme.12116

Type 2 Diabetes: Etiology and Reversibility. Taylor R. *Diabetes Care* 2013; 36: 1047–105. https://care.diabetesjournals.org/content/36/4/1047.full-text.pdf

Weight loss decreases excess pancreatic triacylglycerol specifically in type 2 diabetes. Steven, S., et al. *Diabetes Care* 2016; 39(1): 158–65. https://www.ncbi.nlm.nih.gov/pubmed/26628414

Very low-calorie diet and 6 months of weight stability in type 2 diabetes: Pathophysiologic changes in responders and nonresponders. Steven, S., et al. *Diabetes Care* 2016 May 39(5): 808–15. https://care.diabetesjournals.org/content/early/2016/02/24/dc15-1942

Durability of a primary care-led weight-management intervention for remission of type 2 diabetes: 2-year results of the DiRECT open-label, cluster-randomized trial. Lean, M.E.J., et al. *Lancet Diabetes and Endocrinology* 2019; 7: 344–55. https://www.ncbi.nlm.nih.gov/pubmed/30852132

Remission of human type 2 diabetes requires decrease in liver and pancreas fat content but is dependent upon capacity for beta cell recovery. Taylor, R., et al. *Cell Metabolism* 2018 Oct 2;28(4):547-556. https://reader.elsevier.com/reader/sd/pii/S1550413118304467?token=24A60487ACF5A2C365137132BA2B56D1C27FD40C5F992BEB9B0D38BD89CC0157E871764DE06116F375A5E6705763431C

Understanding the mechanisms of reversal of type 2 diabetes. Taylor, R., et al. *Lancet Diabetes and Endocrinology* 2019; 7: 726–736. https://www.ncl.ac.uk/magres/research/diabetes/reversal/#scientificinformation

Chapter 6

Type 2 diabetes and the diet that cured me. Richard Doughty. https://www.theguardian.com/lifeandstyle/2013/may/12/type-2-diabetes-diet-cure

Normal weight individuals who develop type 2 diabetes: the personal fat threshold. Taylor, R., & Holman, R. *Clinical Science* 2015 Apr;128(7): 405–410. http://www.clinsci.org/content/ppclinsci/128/7/405.full.pdf

Intensive blood-glucose control with sulphonylureas or insulin compared with conventional treatment and risk of complications in patients with type 2 diabetes (UKPDS 33). UK Prospective Diabetes Study (UKPDS) Group. *Lancet* 1998; 352: 837–53. https://www.thelancet.com/action/showPdf?pii=S0140-6736%2898%2907019-6

Integrative genomic analysis implicates limited peripheral adipose storage capacity in the pathogenesis of human insulin resistance. Lotta, L.A., et al. *Nature Genetics* 2017; 49: 17–26. https://www.nature.com/articles/ng.3714.pdf

Diet, lifestyle, and the risk of type 2 diabetes mellitus in women. Hu, F.B., et al. *New England Journal of Medicine* 2001; 345: 790–97

Beta-Cell lipotoxicity in the pathogenesis of non-insulin-dependent diabetes mellitus of obese rats: impairment in adipocyte-B-Cell relationships. Lee, Y. et al. 1994. *Proceedings of the National Academy of Science of U.S.A.* 91: 10878–10882. https://www.ncbi.nlm.nih.gov/pmc/articles/PMC45129/pdf/pnas01145-0129.pdf

Chapter 7

Acceptability of a very-low-energy diet in Type 2 diabetes: patient experiences and behavior regulation. Rehackova, L., et al. *Diabetic Medicine* 2017; 34: 1554–1567. https://www.ncl.ac.uk/magres/research/diabetes/reversal/#scientificinformation

Population response to information on reversibility of type 2 diabetes. Steven, S., et al. *Diabetic Medicine* 2013 Apr; 30(4): e135–8. https://www.ncbi.nlm.nih.gov/pubmed/23320491

Chapter 8

The 8-Week Blood Sugar Diet. Mosley, M. Short Books 2015

The 8-Week Blood Sugar Diet Recipe Book. Bailey, C. Short Books 2016

The Hairy Dieters Make It Easy. King, S. & Myers, D. Seven Dials 2018

Population adiposity and climate change. Edwards P & Roberts I. *International journal of epidemiology*, 38 (4): 1137–40 https://doi.org/10.1093/ije/dyp172

Making China safe for Coke: how Coca-Cola shaped obesity science and policy in China. Greenhaugh, T. *British Medical Journal* 2019; 364: k5050. https://www.bmj.com/content/bmj/364/bmj.k5050.full.pdf

Bibliography

Chapter 9

Hormone Replacement Therapy and Heart Disease Prevention Experimentation Trumps Observation. Petitti, DB. *JAMA*. 1998; 280(7): 650–652. https://jamanetwork.com/journals/jama/article-abstract/187868

Low-energy diets differing in fiber, red meat and coffee intake equally improve insulin sensitivity in type 2 diabetes: a randomised feasibility trial. Nowotny, B., et al. *Diabetologia* 2015; 58: 255–64. https://link.springer.com/content/pdf/10.1007%2Fs00125-014-3457-8.pdf

Goodlad RA 2001 Dietary Fiber and the risk of colorectal cancer. https://gut.bmj.com/content/gutjnl/48/5/587.full.pdf

The Hawthorne studies-a fable for our times? Gale E. *Quarterly Journal of Medicine* 2004; 97: 439–49. https://academic.oup.com/qjmed/article/97/7/439/1605689

Randomized trials in context: practical problems and social aspects of evidence-based medicine and policy. Pearce, W., et al. *Trials* 2015; 16: 394–401. https://www.ncbi.nlm.nih.gov/pmc/articles/PMC4560875/pdf/13063_2015_Article_917.pdf

Snake Oil. Diamond, J. Vintage 2001.

Dietary cholesterol and cardiovascular disease: a systematic review and meta-analysis. Berger, S., et al. *American Journal of Clinical Nutrition* 2015; 102: 276–94. https://pdfs.semanticscholar.org/6e04/1243158a6947441ed1de248855b40c6ad90f.pdf?_ga=2.242082114.1180311127.1564751770-864389371.1564751770

Dietary Saturated and Trans Fatty Acids: Is It Time to Change Track? Astrup, A., et al. *British Medical Journal* 2019; 365: l4137. https://www.bmj.com/content/366/bmj.14137

The Misuse of Meta-analysis in Nutritional Research. Barnard, N.D., et al. *Journal of the American Medical Association* 2017; 318: 1345–36. https://jamanetwork.com/journals/jama/article-abstract/2654401

The Challenge of Reforming Nutritional Epidemiological Research. Ioannidies, J.P.A. *Journal of the American Medical Association* 2018; 320: 969–70. https://jamanetwork.com/journals/jama/article-abstract/2698337

Breakfast is a Dangerous Meal. Kealey T. 4th Estate, London 2016

Belief Beyond the Evidence: Using the Proposed Effect of Breakfast on Obesity to Show 2 Practices to Distort Scientific Evidence. Brown, A.W., et al. *American Journal of Clinical Nutrition* 2013; 98: 1298–1308. https://www.ncbi.nlm.nih.gov/pmc/articles/PMC3798081/pdf/ajcn9851298.pdf

Fruit, vegetable, and legume intake, and cardiovascular disease and deaths in 18 countries (PURE): a prospective cohort study. Miller, V., et al. *Lancet* 2017; 390(10107): 2037–2049. https://www.sciencedirect.com/science/article/pii/S0140673617322535?via%3Dihub

Index

Index

Index

Index

Index

Index

Index

Index

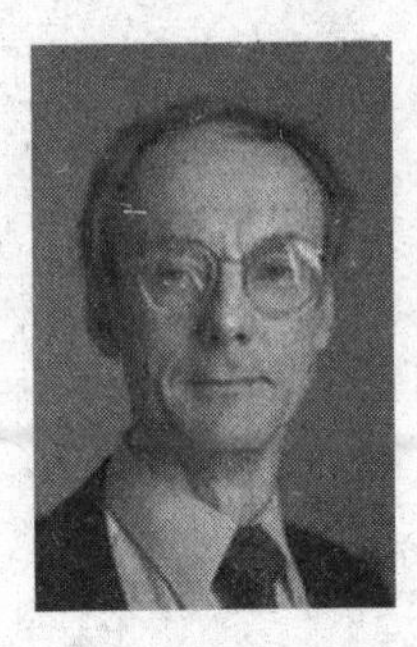

Roy Taylor is professor of Medicine and Metabolism at Newcastle University and Honorary Consultant Physician at Newcastle upon Tyne Hospitals NHS Foundation Trust. He qualified in medicine at the University of Edinburgh. He was visiting professor of medicine at Yale University, USA (1990–91) where he acquired new MRI methods to look into the human body. On returning to the UK he raised £5.2 million to establish the Newcastle MR Centre. He also developed the UK system for screening of diabetic eye disease and is the author of over 300 scientific papers.